POOK'S CAREGIVER

Five Years Coping With

Parkinson's

Lewy Body

Stroke

AFIB

By

Jim Haugen

Copyright Page

Copyright © 2010 by Jim Haugen

All rights reserved. No part of this publication may be reproduced, distributed, or transmitted in any form or by any means, including photocopying, recording, or other electronic or mechanical methods, without the prior written permission of the publisher, except in the case of brief quotations embodied in critical reviews and certain other noncommercial uses permitted by copyright law.

Table of Contents

YEAR 2010 – POOK'S PARKINSON'S DISEASE SHOWS UP

Chapter 1 – An Optimistic Start to the Year

Chapter 2 – A Surprising Call

Chapter 3 - Two PD Diagnoses and Medications

Chapter 4 – PD Doctor Communications

Chapter 5 – Her Year's Health Impacts

Chapter 6 – Caregiver Lesson's learned

YEAR 2011 – AFIB AND LEWY BODY DEMENTIA BEGIN

Chapter 7 – Hip Surgery Leads to AFIB

Chapter 8 – Adding a Lewy Body Dementia Diagnosis

Chapter 9 – My Caregiver Actions

Chapter 10 – Combined AFIB and LBD Treatments – and Fun

Chapter 11 – November Doctor visits

Chapter 12 – Her Health Impacts

Chapter 13 – Caregiver Lessons Learned

YEAR 2012 – COPING WITH HEALTH COMPLEXITY

Chapter 14 – Extending 2011 Knowledge and Capabilities

Chapter 15 - PD Doctor Communications

Chapter 16 – Caregiving Gets More Complex

Chapter 17 – Summer Activities

Chapter 18 – Parkinson's Online Course

Chapter 19 - Doctor Communications and a Research Study

Chapter 20 – Moving From Summer into Winter

Chapter 21 – Her Health Impacts

Chapter 22 – Caregiver Lessons Learned

YEAR 2013 - A SEVERE STROKE HAPPENS

Chapter 23 – Beginning Directions

Chapter 24 – Her Stroke and Experiencing Inpatient Treatment

Chapter 25 – My Post-Stroke Caregiver Actions

Chapter 26 – Experiencing Outpatient Services

Chapter 27 – Doctor Appointments and Results

Chapter 28 – Home Therapy and an Important Reference

Chapter 29 – Another Change in Direction

Chapter 30 – Her Health Impacts

Chapter 31 – Caregiver Lessons Learned

YEAR 2014 – A SHORTENED GOOD-BYE TIME

Chapter 32 – A Renewed Optimistic Direction

Chapter 33 – A Typical Winter Day

Chapter 34 – Doctor Communications and Directions

Chapter 35 - My Changed Caregiver Attitude

Chapter 36 – Pook's Last Months

Dedication

This book is dedicated to our children: Jimmy, Kari, Jan and Leigh –

And to our grandchildren: Laura, Matt, Jamie, Luke, Jake, Nick, Mitch, Kyle, Tyler, Hannah, Kristen, Danny, Maria, and Michael –

With the hope that they will never have to cope with Parkinson's Disease or Lewy Body Dementia inherited from their mom or grandma.

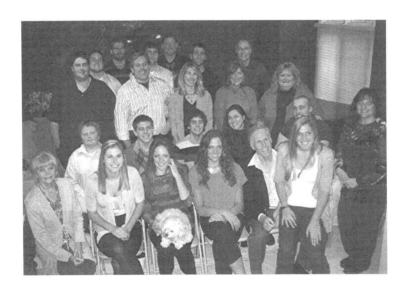

PREFACE

The purpose of this book is to provide helpful information for other patients and caregivers dealing with Parkinson's disease, Lewy Body Dementia, Stroke, Atrial Fibrillation, or similar medical problems, by detailing almost five years of caregiving efforts, and lessons learned, by Pook's caregiver husband, Jim

Prologue

I look for a lost piece of paper in my messy den,
Happen across an envelope of pictures,
A hiking trip to Banff five years previous,
Rush downstairs to reminisce with my wife, Mary Ellen (Pook):
> A treacherous hike along a rocky streambed,
> Clicking rocks noisily together, avoid surprising a grizzly bear,
> Climb along a steep canyon wall, a rushing waterfall at the top,
> Take her picture with a surprising little chipmunk,
> Met halfway up, she's feeding it peanuts,
> Another, the two of us standing side by side, Banff far below us,
> Taken by a friendly European couple on another trail,
> She, lounging on a log, a gorgeous blue-green lake backdrop.

I recall details, now become foggy in her mind,
Still we share a pleasant hour, reliving those days.

A poem, by Dante, sums up what's happened:
"Midway upon the journey of life,
I found myself within a forest dark,
For the straightforward path had been lost".

Our planned future together has drastically changed,
We used to talk and laugh about passing into our eighties,
When we'd be relaxing side-by-side in our rockers.
But, after 56 years together, she now has Parkinson's disease (PD),

And, closely related, Lewy Body Dementia (LBD).
Three years ago tremors began in her right hand,
Additional symptoms soon disrupted her everyday life:
    Paying and balancing the checkbook
    Cooking with well-practiced recipes
    Driving and navigating
    Conversational skills gone
    Her bouncy, smiling personality disappeared

A University of Michigan specialist prescribes,
Helpful Sinemet pills plus Aricept,
Advises daily exercise, physical and mental,
To slowdown any future declines.

I recall a now poignant song from the fifties:
"Those were the days my friend,
We thought they'd never end,
We'd sing and dance forever and a day ----"

Our active lifestyles, now forever left behind:
Travels, outdoor activities and socializing with friends,
Vigorous tennis games; U.S. and overseas trips:
    Club Med, Captiva Island, Kauai,
    Australia's Barrier Reef, Palm Springs ----
Challenging hikes: –
    Mount Manadnock, top of the Breckenridge chairlift,
        Canada's Banff,
    Summer at Vail, Sedona red rocks, New Mexico
        mushroom hunting ----
Downhill skiing: –
    Alpine Valley, Snowmass, Vail, Steamboat, and Tahoe,
    Winter Park, Jackson Hole, Whistler/Blackcomb ----
She collected 250 magnets from these places and activities,

And much, much more.

Beatle's lyrics express it so well –
"Yesterday, all my troubles seemed so far away,
Now it looks as though they're here to stay,
Oh, I believe in yesterday".

Our yesterdays were calendar driven,
Targeting such as the above experiences,
Now, driven by health considerations,
We plot new directions in our lives -
An emphasis on fighting to maintain her capabilities,
New kinds of physical exercises –
    Water aerobics
    Group stretch and strength hours
    Yoga trials
    Dumb-bell workouts
    Bicycling, now peddling a tandem
We add a mental exercise program - –
    Learning poetry
    Reading passages out loud
    Spelling words frontwards and backwards
    Gin rummy and puzzles
Private moments of fun, despite her limitations -–
    Casual walks in the sun
    Laughing about our mental mistakes
    My struggles at replacing her cooking skills
    Visits with our four kids and 14 grandkids
I choke up several times each day,
Seeing her as she is; and how she used to be,
Thankful for what we still have.

I hold onto hope so eloquently phrased by Micron:
"Hope is a dream, one that never ends,

Hope is a friend, one never leaves,
Hope is love, sweet and fragile,
Hope is a door that never closes,
Hope is you and me, what we want our life to be".

I begin a hopeful Internet search for a medical miracle,
Learn more about Parkinson's disease -
Basic research now finds two separate Parkinson networks,
One for movement, one for cognition,
With similarities in Parkinson's with Dementia (PDD),
Alzheimer's (AD) and Lewy Body Dementia (LBD),
All sharing problems with amyloid plaques in the brain.
A cancer drug reverses those amyloid plaques in mice,
A first trial with humans about to begin;
A synthetic version of curry spice also effective on mice,
More human trials yet to begin;
A new drug improves blood flow in stroke victims,
May halt the progression of brain plaques,
Human trials two to three years away;
New gene therapy, injected directly into the brain,
Bypasses the blood-brain barrier, just mild improvements;
Eli Lilly & Medtronic combine to deliver a chemical,
Directly into the brain; potential use years away;
How soon might real miracle solutions appear?

Patti Davis has written a book about her ex-President dad,
Ronald Reagan, and his long bout with Alzheimer's,
Titled "The Long Goodbye", referencing a Dylan Thomas poem:
"Do not go Gentle into that good night,
Old age should burn and rage at close of day,
Rage, rage against the dying of the light."

We, like millions of others, join a race; one of worry versus hope,
I worry about a future of gradually deteriorating symptoms -
> Increasing stiffness; a shuffling walk
> Worsening tremors
> Symptoms spreading to both sides of her body
> Difficulties eating and swallowing
> Medications losing effectiveness
> Her mind gradually deteriorating
> Till she forgets who I am

Remaining positive, I also hope for a timely medical breakthrough -
> Pills that attacks those nasty tangles in her brain
> Her neurons magically restored
> Much of her memory returning
> She regains a bubbling personality
> We laugh that she's just been away for a while"
> We move ahead, resuming old activities

This powerful, important race regarding her health -
The hope of winning means years of anxiety ahead.

I listen to Time in a Bottle by Jim Croce,
Which so well captures my love for her: -
> "If I had a box just for wishes,
> And dreams that had never come true,
> The box would be empty,
> Except for the memory,
> Of how they were answered by you".

My heart goes out to other progressive disease sufferers,
Patients with PD, LBD, AD, or such, and their hopeful caregivers.
I look forward to a day when survivors of these diseases,

Celebrate their recoveries, like cancer survivors - Pook among them.

Description

This book covers three interacting stories – (1) My wife, Pook, and her health deterioration over a period of more than four years; (2) My caregiver efforts during that time, and (3) Problems encountered in confronting the American health system.

1. THE THREE STORIES

Story One – Pook as a patient – Describes her bouts with Parkinson's Disease, Lewy Body Dementia, Stroke, and Atrial Fibrillation; how each of these health problems created major changes in her personality, communication abilities, and physical activities. It also depicts her responses to the numerous different rehabilitation efforts by her husband and other medical personnel.

Story Two – Husband Jim's caregiver efforts – Describes the extended period of time I spent caring for Pook. Above all, it describes my singular fight, beyond the limitations of pills, to withstand the attacks of her progressive diseases, attempting to retain her mental and physical abilities as long as possible – to keep her wonderful personality alive. In the case of her stroke, to attempt to reverse its impacts - restore her ability to walk, and to again be able to use both of her hands. I also: (1) characterize my "lessons learned" as I became educated in the work of a caregiver, as her health was impacted by each problem – her PD, LBD, Stroke, and AFIB; (2) explicitly detail my written communications with her doctors, therapists, family and friends; and (3) cover the nature, benefits and limitations of efforts by other medical personnel as I endeavored to work with them.

Story Three – Confronting the American health system – Describes the nature, strengths and weaknesses of the American health system surrounding Pook – doctors, therapists, systems, facilities and equipment, finances – as they had such important impacts on decisions to maintain, and attempt to rehabilitate, her health. I especially emphasize the lack of honesty, and weaknesses of, the government driven Medicare based approach to stroke rehabilitation.

2. CAREGIVER LESSONS LEARNED

Caregiving is tough, complicated and mentally taxing! Over the course of almost five years as Pook's caregiver, I've learned a lot about the nature of the caregiver's job. Throughout the book you will find references to "My Caregiving Learning Process" describing examples as they apply to different parts of her health situation. Important "lessons learned" from my experiences are outlined below in the hope that you might find them helpful references for working with your patient.

1. Find the "right" medical personnel – especially specialist physicians, and

therapists, with the credentials, and experience, that fit your patient's health situation; including the value of getting second opinions.

2. Establish written communications with medical personnel, as well as with family and friends; they will deeply appreciate seeing status and issues information in writing.

3. Build an understanding of the nature of the medical system you're dealing with – the financial, time, approach, and medical personnel aspects as related to the quality of care your patient receives.

4. Become the "disease fighter" leader in helping your patient work on important actions, such as specific exercise routines, going well beyond just taking pills.

5. Build an understanding of your patient's needs to cope with the negative impacts of his or her diseases and other health problems.

6. Establish goals and action plans, covering durations of several months or more which, if successful, will provide meaningful improvement in your patient's health.

7. Search for, define, and purchase, extra equipment which will aids in your patient's recovery; some of which will involve personal risk taking about their eventual effectiveness.

8. Always convey an optimistic view to your patient, describing how what "we" are doing that will have positive health results.

9. Find a "sitter"/companion to replace you for hours at a time, several days a week;

one with a bouncy temperament that your patient will always look forward to seeing.

10. Always search for new and innovative ideas that, when implemented, will enhance your patient's quality of life.

11. Continually search the Internet for hopeful information regarding developments in better medications or cure for your patient; convey hope.

12. Develop your own personal discipline, patience, and stamina, to be able to prioritize, including multi-tasking, seemingly less important essentials.

13. Implement your own personal approach to maintaining records of your patient's progress and/or setbacks, including tracking periodic changes in medications.

14. Build up and/or maintain your own physical health as needed for daily work with your patient, especially for a time when extensive lifting and movement might be required, with fear of dropping him or her.

15. Keep your hands clean, especially after outside contact, to avoid transmitting flu germs and other possibilities.

3. CAREGIVER MULTI-TASKING ESSENTIALS

It seems, to the caregiver, that there are always too many little jobs to think about and get done each day. Yet fitting these sorts of tasks into each day takes away so much energy that you must keep yourself in good physical condition, or have a lot of daily assistance. Here's a list of many of those "small" things that a caregiver has to somehow fit into daily, weekly, and monthly routines:

Arrange pills for the week; give out pills every four hours; contact Drs. about changing pills

Purchase supplies, such as pills, vinyl gloves, personal cleaners for patient, clothes washing liquid, paper – napkins, toilet paper, towels, waterproof bed under-pads, furnace filters

Adjust settings, load and empty clothes washer, dishwasher, dryer, microwave, oven

Patient personal care – Select clothes, dress and undress, shower and shampoo, tint hair, trim finger and toe nails, comb hair, get haircut, brush teeth, track blood pressure and blood density

Caregiver's own personal care

Adapt house temperature – furnace setting, air conditioning setting, windows open and close

Adjust TV and music settings

Clean house – kitchen, bathroom, rug and carpets, tile floor, dust, spots on floor and rug/carpets, oven, microwave, table tops

Plan and cook meals, purchase food

Move patient in/out bed, various chairs and wheelchair, to/from tables, in/out of car, in/out of buildings

Pay bills, go to bank, balance checkbook and savings account, watch finances

Find time for occasional naps, make lists

Service car

Maintain the house – inside, like air annual filters; and outside, from painting to mowing the lawn or clearing side walk and driveway after snow falls (Fortunately, we were residents of a condo)

ABOUT THE AUTHOR

As Pook's health began to deteriorate, I was fortunate to possess personal characteristics helpful to assuming caregiver responsibilities – a strong educational background; physically fit and energetic for my age (77 years old); retired with lots of time available; living in a condo with minimum maintenance needs; married for 55 years, and deeply in love with Pook; plus a determination that I would never place her in a nursing home. Importantly, I was also lacking in skills that I would have to learn about along the way – knowing little or nothing about medicine and nursing; operation of household appliance; shopping, cooking, washing clothes, vacuuming and otherwise taking care of our household and ourselves.

I have a Mechanical Engineering Degree plus Master's Degrees in Civil Engineering and Business. I have extensive analytical and management experience in aerospace, robotics, automobile design and transportation systems; a specialist background in strategic planning, market planning and marketing of technology based systems; a decade of working as an international consultant; comfortable with oral and written communications with a diversity of clients; previously a monthly feature writer for an International magazine.

I have devoted myself full time to taking care of my wife ever since her health problems began within our condo home. I am now 81 years old. Here's a recent picture:

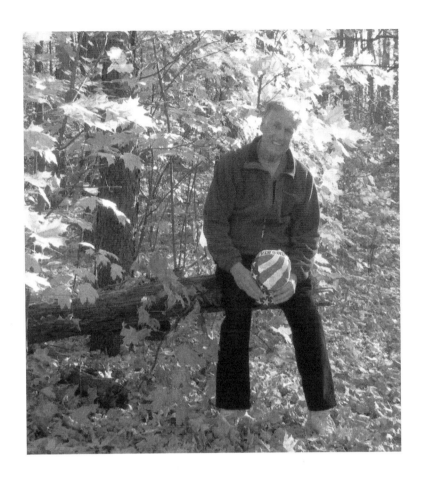

ABOUT POOK

Pook at the time her health began to fail, was 73 years old, had raised four children, and helped with raising 14 grandchildren. She has always been very social, with a friendly outgoing personality; has stayed in great physical condition;

loved the outdoors and physical exercise; enjoyed 30 some years of downhill skiing, tennis, biking, hiking, and, more recently, playing golf. She also played indoor tennis throughout the cold Michigan winters plus going for long walks indoors and out; has retained many friends from tennis, golf and bridge, and continued to get together with them. Many of her activities have been jointly with her husband, considering each other long time best friends.

She has always loved traveling, touring different locales for hiking, skiing and golfing, and for visiting friends and relatives. A number of ship based vacations – ocean going and river cruises – with close friends and relatives were especially highly remembered. Over the years she amassed a collection of refrigerator magnets, each carefully selected for its uniqueness, numbering in excess of 250.

Here are two pictures of her as she looked while still in good health:

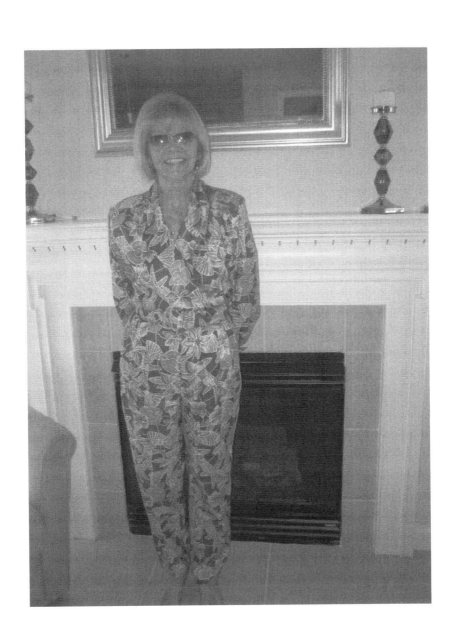

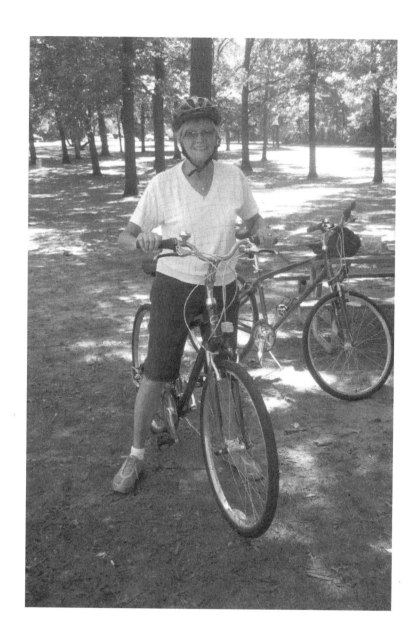

YEAR 2010 – POOK'S PARKINSON'S DISEASE SHOWS UP

CHAPTER 1 – AN OPTIMISTIC START TO THE YEAR

From Summer to Year's End in 2009

Our 2009 summer was filled with our usual activities and we expected that same sort of life to continue throughout 2010:

> Six months of golf – hitting practice balls together and playing golf on different courses, individually with friends and sometimes together.
>
> Many 20 minute bike rides around the small lake we live on; once a week take 40 minute, eight mile long, strenuous bike rides up and down hills at a metro park just 15 minutes away.
>
> A long drive to the Midwest, with both of us sharing the driving, covers almost 3000 miles. We visit relatives on both sides, as well as numerous old friends – good conversations and lots of laughs.

We have a battery powered pontoon boat and spend a delightful Fourth of July on our little lake, watching fireworks, with our daughter and husband and three grandkids.

As fall weather sets in and turns cold, we resume mall walking at a local regional mall as we have done for the previous several years.

We celebrate our 54th anniversary the day after Christmas in 2009 and look forward to more of our usual pleasant fun-filled times in 2010. We already have reservations for the end of January to fly to Mesa, Arizona to visit Pook's sister who has a "snowbird's" house there; also visit Pook's brother and his wife who are permanent residents in Mesa; and see Jim's sister and spouse who have rented a place for several months. While there we will play some golf; go for long walks in the sun; visit the flea market; maybe play some silly, cards, with lots of laugh opportunities; and eat too much going out for lunches and dinners. Additionally, we have made a reservation to rent a house at a golfing community called the Villages in Florida for the month of March.

So we will be shocked by the ensuing health events of 2010

A Worry about Future Health Problems

One afternoon in March, 2009, she drove off to see her doctor some ten miles away. She seemed unusually nervous about her appointment for some reason that she was unable to explain. I'm shocked, when an hour or so later I receive a personal call from her doctor – her pulse rate is over 150, and he will call an ambulance or I can pick her up and take her to the hospital! I rush over and drive her to hospital emergency. The emergency doctor explains how serious her situation is - if they have to chemically intervene to get her heart rate back to normal, she will have to be admitted. He speaks to her in a very calming voice and over a period of 15 or 20 minutes and I watch in amazement as her heart rate gradually returns to normal. Following several additional hours of observation with no pulse rate changes, I'm permitted to take her back home. A later review of heart data is inconclusive as to whether her increased pulse rate was due to atrial fibrillation or a less concerning panic attack.

More Concerns About Future Health Problems

Late in 2009, our two daughters and I discuss some small, noticeable changes in her health – occasionally stumbling over some phrases when in a conversation, and occasional seeing tremors in her right hand. We pretty much discount her talking mistakes as due to "senior citizen moments" that we all occasionally experience, or what is more officially termed "Mild Cognitive Impairment" (MCI). According to a Mayo Clinic Web site:

> "MCI is an intermediate stage between the expected cognitive decline of normal aging and the more serious decline of dementia. It can involve problems with memory, language, thinking and judgment that are greater than normal age-related changes. If you have mild cognitive impairment you may be aware that your memory or mental function has slipped. Family and close friends may notice a change, but generally these changes aren't indications that cognitive impairment may increase your risk of later progression to dementia caused by Alzheimer's disease or other neurological conditions. Some people with mild cognitive impairment never get worse, and a few eventually get better".

We collectively feel that the conversation "slips" we've seen aren't that seriously currently, but that we will keep our eye on the possibility that they could get worse.

I research her right hand tremors and they appear to be "essential tremors" which only happen when she's attempting to use that right hand for some heavy lifting or some fine movements. I notice that while putting on and removing makeup she doesn't exhibit any such tremors. I understand that Parkinson's tremors, in contrast, are expected to occur when a person is resting. So I discount the possibility that she has Parkinson's based on this simplistic view of defining Parkinson's just by the kind of tremors she's experiencing. But I also begin to worry because an older brother of hers had Parkinson's for 12 years and had died from it just a few years previous.

CHAPTER 2 – A SURPRISING CALL

In mid-January, 2010 we receive the kind of early morning call that everyone dreads - our daughter-in-law calls from Florida about our eldest son, Jimmy. She had brought him to a hospital emergency room because he was suffering intense back pain and had been for some time. An initial x-ray of his lower back was negative and the doctor's diagnosis was just a strain, and muscle relaxants prescribed. She insisted on a review by a second doctor who had an x-ray of his upper back taken - showing a huge tumor eating away at his spine. She tells us that he is in the process of being been helicoptered to a research hospital in Gainesville, associated with the University of Florida. He will undergo emergency surgery ASAP in an attempt to save his life. We are both extremely broken up; fly out the next morning, worrying throughout that flight about whether he will make it through the surgery. We arrive while his surgery is still ongoing, then, later in the day, are able to see him briefly in the intensive care unit after he awakens. He is lying there very pale, breathing oxygen with various tubes in his arms connected to bags of dripping fluids. We go through several anxious days while he remains in intensive care, before we return home.

Pook is especially shocked seeing him in such serious condition, has trouble sleeping and resorts to sleeping pills. Her tremors become noticeability more frequent and larger, but are still predominantly occurring during use of her right hand and arm.

Our Continuing 2010 Activities

Despite these new worries, we are committed to fly to Arizona some two weeks later, which turns out to be a needed diversion. Our son is out of the hospital and in post-surgery therapy. We talk to him on the telephone and he provides assurances that he is already doing well with his recovery. Furthermore, he indicates that the doctor in charge of his case feels that, based on initial tests, he doesn't have multiple myeloma, but, rather, much less serious solitary myeloma. So we enjoy our visits with relatives in Mesa. Pook is heavily involved in cooking, with lots of laughter between her and her sister as they prepare dinners for guests. Having left the snow and cold of the Detroit area behind for a while, we relish being in the sunshine and warm temperatures – practice and play golf, with Pook being cheered on by residents adjacent to the golf course when she birdies one hole, a rare occurrence. We go for long walks; tour a flea market and are able to generally relax for the two weeks we are there.

Pook's tremors have seemingly disappeared in this friendly, relaxed, environment; her conversations seemingly normal, with smiles and laughter like old times.

Two months later we make our planned drive to Florida. We will be hosting my sister and husband for the first two weeks of our month's stay, so Pook is focused on menus and recipes in advance of our departure, planning meals to serve our company. We have been assured ahead of the trip that our son's recovery therapy, now as an outpatient, is going well, so his wife would prefer that we delay our visit for a month when he will have completed his in-patient therapy. We share the driving on the way down as we've always done on long trips, changing drivers every hour or so. She drives with no problems, despite encountering heavy traffic in new construction areas several times.

Our company's two week visit is a great diversion, as she is kept busy making most breakfasts and many dinners. We jointly play golf from time to time with; tour the Villages; and make a one day visit to Disney Epcot. St. Patrick's Day occurs while we're at the Villages and we find it to be a big event with a long parade of decorated golf carts. A picture taken there shows Pook and I seated in front of the Villages pond and waterfall now dyed green for the occasion. Dance bands play in the evening and Pook and I go out on the dance floor for one slow and one fast dance. I will later recognize, with deepest sadness, that this is the last time we will ever dance again together!

Another Worry about Future Health Problems

Pook struggles with periodic pain in her leg or hip, sometimes attributed by her to a possible groin pull incurred earlier while playing winter indoor tennis. I wrap her upper thigh with an elastic wrap every time we are going out to play golf, and it seems to help.

After our company departs, we are by ourselves a lot and Pook is distraught and worried about what sort of condition our son will be in when we stop by his house to see him and his wife, following completion of his therapy. This thought is obviously weighing heavily on her mind. In the interim, we socialize with an old friend of Pook's and her husband. She and her friend have a long-time history of tennis and golf together. We play golf, go out to restaurants several times and otherwise socialize. Pook's participation in discussions has become noticeably subdued compared to her usual outgoing personality.

The Trauma of Visiting Our Son

I do all the driving for the four hours it takes to arrive at our son's house. I offer to let her also drive, as usual, but she is very distraught about our forthcoming visit and refuses. When we arrive, he is sitting outside, waiting to great us. We follow him in, his slow, shaky walking ability readily apparent. I'm pleased to see him doing this well after all he has gone through. Pook again is mostly quiet. He speaks openly about his condition – his surgery has left parts of his legs and body partially numb; his back, where metal supports have replaced lost vertebrae, makes it difficult to sit in one position for long periods, and hinders his sleeping. He is optimistic about further progress as he works out on his own, looking forward to ever longer walks and returning to riding a bike in the near future. We stay for only about an hour, as he still tires easily.

Pook's Health Deterioration

Pook is shocked to finally visit our son and talk about his health condition, especially seeing how badly he walks, and hearing about continuing numbness in parts of his legs. This has a huge depressing impact on Pook's behavior. After we leave, she expresses her concerns about whether he will ever walk normally again; ever be able to resume work; ever have a return of his Multiple Myeloma cancer. She refuses to share in the driving for the remainder of the trip home, talks very little, and spends the majority of the time curled up and sleeping against the passenger side door. After we arrive back home, I am very concerned about how her health has been changing, so begin writing a daily journal. Some of my observations:

> She has begun looking very elderly, with her normal expressive face somewhat frozen in appearance
> The tremors in her right hand keep getting worse
> Her conversational ability is maybe only one quarter of normal in a group setting
> She has stiffened up somewhat and has slowed down a lot
> She has forgotten many normal everyday things, like details about hockey games; despite both of us being long time Red Wings fans
> She tells me that she feels "discombobulated"
> I worry about whether she might have had a small stroke
> We try playing tennis one afternoon, but quickly quit as she can no longer run after balls and has lost most of her coordination for swinging at the tennis balls

We routinely go for regular two mile walks as we have done for years and go for half hour bike rides, despite her continuing leg pain. I frequently wrap an elastic bandage around her upper thigh to minimize her pain

We hit some practice golf balls and she still drives to several golf courses to play golf with her lady friends, using a golf cart all the time

One or two evenings a week we play ping pong, a long-term source of enjoyment. She has always been a good aggressive player, but is noticeably stiff when bending to pick up a ball off the floor.

She spends increasing amounts of time sitting and reading

She sleeps poorly, complains about restless legs, gets up in the middle of the night frequently, to go downstairs and fall asleep on the couch; takes sleep aids frequently.

My Caregiver Actions

I make an appointment to see our family doctor. He gives her the usual general physical tests and the results all come back positive within a few days. Her basic health is fine, but he recommends she see a neurologist about her tremors. I've always been a believer in the importance of written communications, so begin what will prove to be my general approach to all of her doctor visits, preparing a written situation note for the neurologist to review at our meeting:

Dear Neurologist:

Mary Ellen Haugen has always been in great health and is very athletic – tennis, golf, biking, hiking, long daily walks and even ping pong, all of which continue at this time. She has always been very social through her bridge group, tennis and golf groups, plus maintaining contact with neighbors and our 14 grandkids.

In January of 2006 she slipped on the ice and broke her left wrist, requiring surgery and the installation of a metal insert. In January of this year, our son was diagnosed with a rare form of cancer and required immediate surgery to save his life. We flew down to Florida and spent several days waiting through his surgery and follow-up. She has taken this ordeal, which continues, very hard, sometimes waking at night worrying about him. She doesn't sleep well at night and routinely complains about only getting four or five hours of sleep.

Sometime during the past year or so, we both have noticed these symptoms of decline in her health:

Essential tremors have begun in her right hand (occurring while handling something a bit heavy or requiring precision movement, but not occurring while at rest).

Some of her movements seem slow and stiff

She feels different mentally, and even her kids have noticed that she isn't as conversational and experiences lapses in her understanding

She has begun to worry about her own health

I have these specific concerns:

Could she have had a small stroke during the past year? (Even though her blood pressure periodically tested at home, is always below normal – typically like 105/63)?

Does she have some basic physical problem or chemical deficiency causing these symptoms?

We worry about the possibility of Parkinson's disease, since her older brother died from that about two years ago.

CHAPTER 3 – TWO PD DIAGNOSES AND MEDICATIONS

The Neurologist's Examination and Result

The neurologist examines her physically and mentally for about 15 minutes and schedules an MRI. At a second appointment he reviews the MRI results with us, saying that it shows no evidence of her having a brain tumor or having had a stroke. He then states his diagnosis - she does have Parkinson's disease. We had been preparing ourselves for this possibility, but hoping that he will have found some other underlying cause for her health deficiencies. He prescribes a new drug called AZILECT (Rasagiline); provides a prescription and supplies us with some samples.

Returning home we spend several days discussing his diagnosis. Our emphasis is on her brother Bud's bout with PD for some 12 years before dying; also her aunt, Betty, similarly dying from PD. One part of our reaction is "how unfair it is for her to get PD". She has always taken such good care of herself, eating the right foods, staying in good physical condition, in contrast to the lifestyles of several of her brothers. Our second reaction is "research hope" -

surely the continuing medical research on PD since her brother died, and the ongoing research to be completed in the next five or 10 years will result in better medications and possibly a cure.

My Continuing Caregiver Actions

I review articles about diagnosing Parkinson's disease and find information about how difficult it is to diagnose, since no one specific testis available to prove whether a person has it or not. The "usual" signs and symptoms of PD may have other causes, such as dementia with Lewy Bodies and other sources. It is especially difficult to diagnose in the early stages, when at least two of the four main symptoms must be present:

   Tremors or shaking

   Bradykinesia, slowness of movement

   Rigidity, stiffness of arms or legs

   Postural instability

Yes, she has the first two of those symptoms, though her tremors are suspect since they don't usually occur while she's at rest.

The drug the neurologist prescribes is new, only on the market for about six months, and is very expensive; it is marketed as not only assisting in control of PD symptoms but also having preventive capabilities to keep PD from getting worse. I proceed to research the drug on the Internet. The basis for the use of Rasagiline, and its supposed preventive capabilities, is a study called 'The Adagio Study". A Professor Olanow, co-principal investigator, comments on the study: "The ADAGIO Study, the first of its kind, was prospectively designed to demonstrate if AZILECT can slow down the progression of Parkinson's disease. Results of the study show that early treatment, with once daily 1 mg Rasagiline tablets, provided significant clinical benefits that were not obtained by those patients where initiation of AZILECT therapy was delayed by nine months". This sounds like a breakthrough drug and Pook's neurologist has apparently accepted its use on this basis.

My review also finds an article critical of the ADAGIO study, written by a member of the Department of Neurology of the Mayo clinic. This article, from Neurology magazine, raises a series of questions as to whether its ability as a so-called "neuroprotective agent" is really proven. I decide to seek a second opinion as to (1) whether she really has Parkinson's and (2) whether AZILECT is the most appropriate medication. I look for information on the University of Michigan website and find that the University has a specialized unit called The Movement Disorders Clinic, staffed by MD's with additional specialized training in movement disorders, such as those associated with PD. I schedule a meeting with a Doctor there for the following week.

The Movement Disorder Specialist's Examination and Results

I supply the second doctor with Pook's background, similar to what I supplied to her original neurologist. Pook is given a thorough and impressive examination during her appointment. Here's a copy of the note that I sent to family members the day after our University of Michigan appointment:

An Improved Parkinson's Health picture

> *We took your mom to the University of Michigan Movement Disorders Clinic yesterday to get a*

second opinion on her Parkinson's disease diagnosis and what a breath of fresh air!!! The doctor, and two other members of his team, spent an unbelievable hour and 45 minutes with us. An MD and an intern spent the first hour taking her through a huge number of motor function maneuvers, moving her fingers, hands, arms, legs and feet through different ranges of motion and strength checks; reflexes checks; wiggling her tongue and moving her eyes around; walking on her heels and toes; checking her balance and recovery from being pulled off-balance; looking at her writing and ability to copy a drawing of a picture; etc. Overall they seemed to be very pleased and surprised with how she performed, having almost no apparent stiffness or range of motion symptoms. They also asked her about a hundred questions about when this all began, how she feels, what are her worst symptoms, etc. The last half hour was spent with the senior staff doctor, also an MD, who said that he spends every day just working with Parkinson's patients, and is very impressive. He took her through some additional checks and observed her walking and balance ability.

The results are:

1. *Based on his experience with PD patients, the doctor feels that she has a mild form of PD. Patients with the mild symptoms she has at the beginning; usually don't have their health deteriorate into really bad Parkinson symptoms later on.*

2. *He recommends a huge emphasis on exercise, exercise - exercise is more important than any medication, and does more to stave off PD health deterioration; also says to make sure to have fun and enjoy life.*

3. *He feels that she probably has Parkinson's, but that will likely take years to officially confirm.*

4. *Her worst symptom is the tremors in her right hand and that is worse when she feels tense and anxious, which is most of the time. He recommended, and gave her a prescription for, an anti-anxiety medication. She is to remain on that for one month to see whether it improves her resting tremors, and, possibly, her sleeplessness.*

5. *He knew a lot about the medication that her previous neurologist has put her on, Azalect (Rasagiline), and felt that its benefits are over-rated. The possibility of it having a neuro-protective effect, that is, delaying the onset of Parkinson's worsening, is hyped by the*

pharmaceutical company, but is essentially not yet proven. He suggested that she might want to try that medication for one month, after she spends the month on the anti-anxiety medication, and then compare how she feels on each, but don't do both at the same time.

6. Her mental processes have just slowed, as expected with Parkinson's, but she has no evidence of dementia or early Alzheimer's.

7. He also prescribes Sinemet (Carbo –Levadopa) which has been used for some 30 or 40 years and is a generic drug, costing only about $ 4.00 per month. He started Pook out taking only a single pill, three times daily – at 8:00 AM, 2:00 PM and 8:00 PM.

Her medication is immediately effective, improving her slowness of movement, and unfreezing her mask face symptoms so that she exhibits more emotions, including smiling much like she did before. It does nothing to improve her tremors however. She began taking the ant-anxiety pills every day and whether they are effective or whether they provide a placebo effect, she has become less anxious. She takes the Rasagiline for one month and experiences no improvement in her symptoms. We schedule a follow-up meeting with her U of M doctor for the first week of October, canceling a follow-up meeting with her original neurologist. I have quickly learned the importance of getting a second opinion.

My Caregiver Actions - Following Her New PD Diagnosis

The pragmatic decision maker side of me takes over, so I begin to plan what actions I need to take to help her:

> I buy the book "Yoga for Dummies" and immediately begin attempting to teach ourselves the basic principles of Yoga. I find it tough to figure out how to do the exercises properly by reading descriptions and following a few simple pictures and diagrams. But I also find an ongoing Yoga program, held on Saturday mornings, about half an hour away, and sign us both up.
>
> I locate an ongoing evening water aerobics program at a local Junior college about half an hour away and enroll us. Pook has always been uncomfortable in the water, so I agree to join her in participating in all sessions.

I also find that a local Parkinson's Research Fair is being held the next weekend and we both eagerly attend. We learn the following:

> We sit next to a Parkinson's patient diagnosed just a year or two earlier, who seems to have no symptoms whatsoever. She tells us about her exercise program which includes yoga and water aerobics; how important she feels it is to learn yoga through an experienced teacher; and how much better she feels since beginning those programs.
>
> We are both shook to see various PD patients exhibiting big differences in current symptoms – some in wheelchairs, some with the shuffling gait so characteristic of the disease that we had previously seen in her brother. We ask ourselves - What will her future be like, and how soon might she begin to show some of the worse symptoms?
>
> Of special interest is a talk about future medications/techniques for Parkinson sufferers. There is no mention of significant breakthrough possibilities on the near-term horizon or possibilities of a cure in the next ten years or so. We are left with the feeling

that the only real hope is stem cell research, still 10 to 20 years away.

Our Revised Activities

Water Aerobics

The wife of a couple of good traveling friends has had leg surgery and been taking water aerobics for conditioning. So I send her the following e-mail about our water aerobics experience:

Dear Rhoda –

Water aerobics isn't for wimps! We had our first session last evening from 7 to 8 and it was tough. There were about 35 people – 30 women and 5 men, spread around the pool at the local community college. We proceeded to learn all about the variety of exercises that you can do in the water to get/keep your body in shape. We spent some time kicking back and forth the length of the pool, using foam covered dumbbells to keep our heads above water; fins to help us keep moving. Then we were subjected to a variety of splashing kicks with our bare feet while hanging on to the pool side gutters. Another exercise was to use the high water resistance dumbbells in a host of different ways – swinging them up and down through the water, frontwards, backwards and sideways. Lastly, we had to place our legs up along the pool-side and perform different exercises, moving our legs up and down, plus pushups, and jumping up out of the water while hanging onto the sides. Needless to say, we were extremely happy when the hour ended, tired but refreshed. We're looking forward to gradually getting in shape and comfortable with all the exercises in the next several weeks. We take our hat off to you as we understand that you do water aerobics three days a week.

Our Yoga Program

The yoga class is meets every Saturday morning and runs for a dozen sessions. The instructor is a young (less than 30 years old) Master's degree college student who has a decade's worth of experience teaching yoga. She turns out to be an excellent and sympathetic instructor. We had previously acquired yoga mats and, being the only place them in a far corner of the room. The lights are kept dim and our instructor speaks to the class in a low soothing voice. She comes around frequently personally correcting our various poses as needed. She also supplies stretching straps for some exercises and lightweight blocks to lessen the extent of certain stretches. We quickly begin adding distinctive terms to our vocabularies - Warrior pose, thunderbolt, cobra and locust postures; downward facing dog, Swiss army knife, etc., depending on which parts of your body you want to work to improve. We learn a series of a dozen postures incorporated into one overall dynamic termed the sun salutation. Pook is so pleased with the relaxed, low key nature of our first day's work out, that she takes the time to convey her personal pleasure in the class to the instructor.

My Caregiver Health

During July I am taken to the hospital two different times with what appears to possibly be a heart attack. A Diagnosis following the second trip is that I am having gallstone attacks and should consider having my gall bladder removed. After again considering two alternative surgeons, I am more comfortable with one I've located at the University of Michigan and have surgery in August. Fortunately, my recovery from surgery takes only a few days and I'm able to do everything necessary to take care of Pook. The experience, however, leaves our kids jittery about "what if" something happens to incapacitate me for a long stretch of time – who will care for their mom?

CHAPTER 4 – PD DOCTOR COMMUNICATIONS

Here's a copy of the handout I prepared for our follow on October meeting with him:

Dear Parkinson's doctor:

> *Medication*
> *She has been taking one Sinemet pill, three times per day since 7/6/10. You originally prescribed an anxiety medication also, but she quit taking that after one month, feeling it was unnecessary.*
>
> *She also takes: one 81 mg aspirin every morning; a Centrum Silver multivitamin; and one Caltrate calcium and vitamin D supplement.*
>
> *Exercise*
> *She walks almost every day, up to one mile, depending on how well she has slept, how tired she is feeling and what the weather is like. She formerly walked two miles frequently, but now is hampered too much with leg pain.*
>
> *She is participating in a formal Yoga class ever Saturday morning for one hour and twenty minutes.*

She is participating in a formal water aerobics class every Monday night for one hour.

She considers both exercise programs difficult and tiring, but plans to continue with both as important to her PD health.

Health Status

The Sinemet has greatly improved her PD symptoms.

She has continuing right leg pain every day, from her hip to knee primarily. On a scale of one to ten, with ten meaning excruciating pain, her leg pain ranges from the two or three level to the eight level. She wakes up every night with leg pain at the eight level after Yoga or aerobics exercise; and, increasingly, during or after walking. She has tried using a heating pad on her leg during the day but feels it doesn't help that much.

She goes to bed at about 11:30 PM; lies on her back with her knees bent to be somewhat comfortable when in bed. She *wakes up most nights between 1:00 AM and 3:00 AM, goes downstairs and attempts to resume sleep on a downstairs sofa. She has tried an over the counter sleep aid called Simply Sleep, but has lately given up on it as ineffective.*

<u>Other medication</u>
She tried taking 1-1/2 Sinemet three times a day for one week; then 2 Sinemet pills similarly for two days, to see if the change might help with her leg pain, but neither approach helped.

She has also tried taking aspirin for leg pain, then changed to Advil, then during the last several days has tried Aleve; none has helped that much.

PD Doctor Response

He agrees that the Sinemet she is taking has improved her PD symptoms significantly

He prescribes: (1) taking two Amitriptyline pills at bedtime to help her sleep; and (2) taking up to two Tramadol during the day for leg pain.

The next week I call him back about her leg pain still being severe and he: (1) prescribes Gabretin for that pain; and (2) sets her up with an EMG for October 19, to determine if she may be having radiated sciatica pain. The sciatica nerve, which extends from the lower back to the buttocks and backs of the legs, can cause symptoms such as tingling, numbness, weakness or shooting pain down a thigh and leg.

Further PD doctor follow-up communications

Her current Situation

1. *Her sleep problems continue. Four days ago she tried taking a dose of Tramadol before going to bed, instead of Amitriptyline. This approach worked great and she is now sleeping about seven hours each night.*

2. *She tried taking Tramadol twice each day for leg pain with not much help. She forced herself to try walking three blocks yesterday and broke down in tears from the leg pain. She has not filled the Gabretin prescription because: (1) fear of further side effects that will add to her periodic confusion; and (2) wanting to get at the source of her pain.*

3. She completed the EMG testing, and the attending doctor indicated the testing showed she did not have Sciatica.

Further Caregiver Actions

I finally contact a hip surgeon regarding having her hip checked. Here's the note I presented to him at our meeting:

Mary Ellen Haugen, Health Situation

Current

She has right leg pain every day and it has been getting worse since mid-September. The pain is in the front upper half of her leg only; sometimes in the groin/hip area; sometimes in the knee; sometimes the entire upper leg. The pain is worse when standing up from a seated position; as she goes to sit down; and when entering or leaving a car. Standing for any length of time aggravates the leg; sitting and lying down help, so she spends most of the day reading. She is only capable of walking maybe 50 feet indoors because of the severity of her leg pain.

She was diagnosed as having Parkinson's disease by a doctor at the University of Michigan Movement Disorders Clinic in July of this year, and began taking Sinemet medication three times a day on July 6. Her doctor prescribed 50 mg Tramadol starting 10/26, because of her leg pain. She began takes one each night at bedtime only, to help her sleep.

History

She has always been athletically active, playing tennis and golf, biking and walking. About a year or so ago, she would periodically complain of feeling groin pain for a few days after some exercise. This became more frequent on a Florida vacation last March, complaining of a burning sensation in her thigh muscle, but wrapped her leg with an elastic bandage and continued to walk nine hole golf courses.

Up until mid-September, she could still walk a mile or more some days. She began a once a week water aerobics program for one hour at that time; and once a week Yoga class for one hour 20 minutes. She discontinued both in mid-October because of the worsening leg pain. We feel the aggressive *water aerobics leg kicking may have caused the worsening leg pain.*

Medications

1. Takes Sinemet 25/100 three times a day for Parkinson's.
2. Discontinued taking Tramadol last Friday because of mental confusion concerns.
3. She is now just taking Aleve to help with her leg pain, but it doesn't help much.

Medical testing

1. She underwent EMG testing at the University of Michigan on 10/29 because of Sciatica concerns. The results were negative for muscle and nerve problems.

Previous Surgery

She had wrist surgery in January of 2009 because of a fall on the ice.

Hip Surgeon's Response

He has an x-ray taken within half an hour and discusses the deterioration of her hip that it shows. He expresses his view that a cortisone shot will eliminate her pain within just a few days, but he can't predict how fast the hip might continue to get worse, so he has no idea how long the cortisone shot will successfully alleviate her pain. She is given the cortisone injection the next day and within three days can walk with no pain and is able to again sleep all night.

Resumption of Normal Activities

I define a simplified yoga stretching program that we do in our basement area, using techniques we learned in our three days of formal lessons. I also add muscle strengthening work using 6 pound dumbbells for her and 12 pound ones for myself. We continue playing golf, separately and together, plus practice hitting golf balls; biking together around our lake and over the tough metro park trails; and continue our almost daily long walks.

With Pook feeling free of pain again, but no longer feeling capable of safely driving on freeways, we elect to take two short trips within Michigan. Each trip to what the locals refer to as "upper Michigan" has us staying overnight. We visit half a dozen small towns, tour their unique shops, eat a variety of restaurants; buy her a nice little dressy sport coat; visit two wineries and buy bottles of their Michigan wines. The trips are completely relaxing with Pook exhibiting almost no Parkinson's symptoms. Several pictures show her smiling broadly, her facial expressions near normal.

With winter due to commence in a few months, we decide to paint and decorate our kitchen/family room in a lighter and more cheerful set of colors. She drives to a number of fabric shops on her own, selecting one red and yellow pattern for new valances. She has trouble resuming use of her twenty year old sewing machine, so we buy a new sewing machine with easy to use features.

We agree on an approach to design and sew window valances. She sews them all in two days and I manage to hang them appropriately. She selects a bright yellow wall color that harmonizes with the valance pattern and I crawl around cabinets getting the walls painted. We then finish up with a few small additions to furniture and are proud to have a very sunny looking room for the winter – never suspecting that this now cheery room, will become her downstairs sleeping room within several years.

CHAPTER 5 – HER HEALTH IMPACTS

The year 2010 will always live in our memories as a year of health surprises; a roller coaster of emotions, living with the uncertainties of the future, and adapting to the restrictions of a modified life-style.

Pook has learned that she has Parkinson's, with high probability, with an approach with good prospects for a cure approach apparently impossible within the next 10 to 20 years. She has seen her brother die from the same disease and must now live emotionally with the uncertainty of what its long-term effects will be on her. For the near term, her daily life will be restricted by the symptoms she is already experiencing – tremors, stiffness and slowness especially. PD has already taken away her ability to continue to play tennis. Fortunately she is able to continue with other forms of enjoyable physical exercise outside – golf, walking, and biking, plus adding new indoor stretching exercising, weights work and yoga. Here's her picture that I took during our trip to northern Michigan.

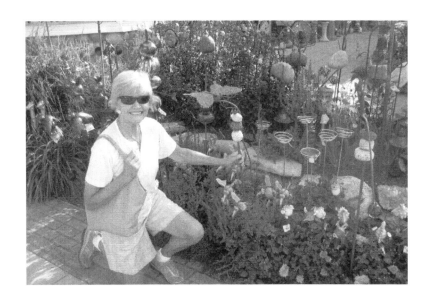

CHAPTER 6 – CAREGIVER LESSON'S LEARNED

I have completed an initial year as Pook's caregiver, learning a lot as I tried various actions. These actions especially turned out to be important:

1. Use written communications, especially with doctors, but also with relatives and with some friends. Pook's doctors commented to me how much they appreciated have background information, her current health status and any questions and issues in writing when we met, and when having any follow on concerns. Pook's children were likewise pleased to learn directly what transpired with doctor visits.

2. The value of obtaining a second opinion, coupled with learning the importance of having access to a Movement Disorder's specialist at a research university; a better selection, because of his daily work with PD patients versus a Neurologist who is spread across patients with much broader health issues.

3. The value of Web research, as demonstrated by my ability to learn about problems with the ADAGIO study; finding out about the Movement Disorders clinic at the University of Michigan.

4. The value of immediate action in starting on exercise to counteract PD symptoms; coupled with the need to be adaptable, as I found out about Pook's personal struggles with formal water aerobics and yoga.

5. Taking care of the caregiver, as I learned I was personally vulnerable, having to have gall bladder surgery.

I also established an implicit first goal, based on discussion with her PD doctor – continue to find daily sources of enjoyment; lead a close to normal life. I found that the more we were able to continue with enjoyable activities, such as sports and a travel, the less anxious, and more relaxed she was, with positive impacts on her tremors and facial muscles.

What will the year 2011 be like as we cope with living with Pook's PD and search for continuing happiness together, despite the change?

YEAR 2011 – AFIB AND LEWY BODY DEMENTIA GET DIAGNOSED

CHAPTER 7 – HIP SURGERY LEADS TO AFIB

I write a Christmas letter to inform all our friends of the good and not so good times of 2010. She is still capable of helping me with getting the cards out; writes brief personal notes to friends on some of them. We bring up all the Christmas decorations from the basement, put out our traditional house decorations, and hang stuff on the Christmas tree. We work side by side doing everything and it's so encouraging to see very little evidence of her Parkinson's, only occasional light tremors. Our daughter hosts the family Christmas Eve celebration, relieving Pook of that burden, and Pook seems like a normal participant in the festivities. We enjoy a quiet celebration by ourselves of our 55th wedding anniversary. Winter weather having set in, she spends a lot of time curled up in a living room chair reading, rarely exhibiting resting tremors. She completes a book at an average of every three or four days. We're busy traveling to the library every week or so, searching lists of books written by her favorite authors to find ones she hasn't read

I wonder how much she understands about each book, so I interrupt her one time and ask a few questions about the book's plot. She can't summarize what a book is all about, as she reads it. However, when I ask her about the particular section she's reading, she's able to describe key characters and what they're doing. From then on I'm content to just let her sit and enjoy her reading.

We also begin winter mall walking – driving to a major regional mall about five miles away. We get there about 9 or 9:30, when the mall doors are unlocked for mall walkers, before the stores open for shoppers. Previous years we have gone there and walked around both floors of the entire inside; once in a while also walking around a third time. We now limit our walk to circling a single floor only once. She is the leader, always setting a fast pace when we begin. We get to know a number of fellow walkers, who show up at about the same time as us, waving or saying "hi" as we pass each other going in different directions. She walks relatively well, at a good pace and with a good arm swing. However, one day, near the end of February, she stops and sits down about half-way around, complaining that her right leg, where she previously had the Cortisone shot, has begun aching. We rest for a while, and then return, more slowly to the beginning and back to the car.

Pook's AFIB Problem Shows up

I schedule a return visit to her same hip surgeon as before. His answer, following another x-ray: No more Cortisone shots. She must now have hip replacement surgery. Following a number of preliminaries, she has that surgery on March 8.

The surgery goes fine that afternoon. However, the next morning I receive an early morning call at home; her heart is in atrial fibrillation, with an erratic heart beat ranging between 150 and 200 beats per minute. A hospital heart specialist prescribes a drug given intravenously which gradually causes her heart beat to return to normal. She is cleared to return home three days later, given a prescription for pills to keep her heart rate slowed down and in rhythm.

One evening, two days later, I check her pulse and she's again in AFI, her heart rate above 125 beats per minute, and I bring her to hospital emergency. I remain there all night, along with two of our children, as her heart doctor remotely monitors the situation, prescribing, as we understand it, several low level doses of Metoprolol, in attempts to restore her heart back to normal rhythm. She remains in AFIB and is re-admitted to the hospital. The next morning the doctor tries applying electrical stimulating "paddles" several times to try to shock her heart back into normal rhythm. His efforts are unsuccessful and her heart remains in AFIB, so he gives her a prescription for a medicine which will allow her heart to remain in AFIB. He then also has the nurse give her Metroprolol, at a higher dose than before. Surprisingly, as Pook is getting ready to leave, we watch the still operating heart monitor, and see her heart return to normal rhythm.

My Caregiver Actions

I begin to research AFIB on the Internet. AFIB is defined as representing a loss of synchrony between the heart's atria and ventricles; characterized as a storm of electrical energy, causing the upper chambers to quiver or fibrillate at high frequency. I also find that AFIB is on the rise, the incidence doubling with each decade of adult life; 10% of the U.S, population over 70 years of age having AFIB. And different types of AFIB exist:

       Lone AFIB with no identifiable cause

Paroxysmal AFIB which occurs intermittently and varies in frequency and duration from a few seconds to several hours or even days

Persistent AFIB which becomes the primary heart rhythm

Adrenergic AFIB that occurs as a result of excessive adrenaline from stimulation of the nervous system, possibly caused by emotional stress or physical exertion.

Treatment involves the use of beta blockers to slow down the heart rate to 70-90 beats per minute, to avoid triggering an AFIB episode, plus taking an anticoagulant or blood thinner such as Coumadin or use of an antiplatelet drug such as aspirin.

An index, termed the CHADS score, has been developed for estimating the risk of stroke in patients with AFIB. The CHAD factors used are:

C – Condition - 1

H – hypertension/blood pressure - 1

A – Age in years - 1

D – Diabetes - 1

S – Stroke prior – 2

For patients with a CHAD score of zero, the annual stroke risk is 1%. For a CHAD score of 1, the annual stroke risk is 2.8%. For patients with a score of 1 (Pook's score), the risk is considered moderate and either aspirin or Coumadin can be used, based on patient preference. Based on this information, I decide to give Pook one 81 mg aspirin every day and a 325 mg aspirin whenever she goes into AFIB.

AFIB Doctor Visits and Communications

Over the course of several meetings with her existing heart doctor I become upset with my inability to hold a reasonable two-way conversation. We have brief meetings in which he dictates his opinions and responds very briefly to any questions from me. He has prescribed a new drug, called Multaq, in addition to a prescription for Metoprolol. The Multaq is for rhythm control; the Metoprolol for rate control. I research Multaq on the Internet and become concerned about its side effects. Multaq has only been marketed for about a year and questions have arisen about severe side effects - causing liver problems and, in several cases, apparent liver failure. I provide our doctor a one and one-half page summary of my research regarding Multaq and possible action:

Mary Haugen, and her husband, would like to make the following prescription changes: (1) immediately quit taking Multaq; and (2) phase out her use of Metropolol over the next week or two, for the following reasons:

Multaq

She has noticed recurring redness, rashes and itching on her arms, side effects possibly related to Multaq use. She is working on controlling this rash by the use of an over-the-counter ointment.
The consumer advocacy group, Public Citizen, has classified Multaq as a do not use drug. They recommend that current users talk to their doctors about getting off it as soon as possible, due to the potential danger of serious liver injury.

I am concerned that only 16 months after Multaq sales were initiated, serious concerns about health consequences are already emerging.

Review of the Athena trial of Multaq use, indicates that Mary is not an appropriate user, based on the following:

> 86% of the trial patients had hypertension and were on two different classes of anti-hypertension drugs, with a mean systolic blood pressure of 134. Mary has always had low blood pressure of about 100/60, without any medication, and has always been very athletic.
> 60% of the trial patients had structural heart defects (Mary has none)
> 60% were taking an oral anti-coagulant such as Coumadin; Mary does not take such a drug.
> Only 6% of the trial patients had lone AFIB like Mary

Dr. Hohnloser, part of the Athena study, sums up the trial limitations by saying: "Future trials should consider patients under 75 without additional cardio-vascular risk factors. The exclusion of these patients from this study limits the application of the results".

Metoprolol

> Mary's AFIB is apparently defined as "lone" type – with no identifiable cause, or having no associated

abnormalities of the heart, (she has none) or –

paroxysmal", occurring intermittently, only having happened after her hip replacement surgery or –

Adrenergic, since it appears to be directly related to the emotional stress/anxiety of her hip replacement surgery

We understood the purpose of the beta blocker she has been taking is to prevent her heart rate from becoming too rapid, preventing AFIB. Her risk of having another AFIB episode is unknown, but may relate to some future episode of emotional stress

We have the following concerns, some of which may be directly related to her use of this drug:

> *Her heart rate is being maintained in a Bradycardia range between about 47*

and 60 beats per minute; a concern as she resumes aerobic exercising. We expect her heart beat to return to its normal resting rate of about 70 beats per minute without medication

She has trouble sleeping and wakes up in the middle of every night

She has a continuing feeling of being "over-medicated"; she is already taking Parkinson's medication which contributes to that same feeling

She exhibits memory lapses and confusion on a daily basis; a possible side effect

> *She fights daily drowsiness episodes*
>
> *We request your assistance in managing her withdrawal from the use of Metoprolol:*
>
> > *Establishing an appropriate rate of reduction in pill size*
> >
> > *Establishing a regimen for monitoring the results during and following withdrawal*
> >
> > *Defining appropriate intervention should her AFIB return*

His response, surprisingly, is to crumple up my notes with only a casual glance at them. He then lectures me about his experience of many years and that I should not, therefore, question his judgment.

My Further Caregiver Actions

This last episode with her AFIB doctor leads me to search for a second opinion. Fortunately the University of Michigan is only a 30 minute drive away from our residence, and we have already been greatly impressed with Pook's Parkinson's doctor. Easy research on the U of M web site leads me to a specialist in AFIB, who is also a researcher in treatments to cure AFIB. We have an appointment with him several weeks later and I supply him a copy of the same material that I had given to her existing AFIB doctor.

His manner is extremely casual and friendly. He reviews her heart data from the hospital, which we have had forwarded to him, and agrees with the diagnosis, that she had been in AFIB. His further response to the previous doctor's comments is jovial. He indicates that we should have suggested that we have a right to question his decisions, since we, through our appointments, are paying his salary. Second, he immediately takes Pook off Multaq, instead wanting her limited to the rate control drug, Metropolol. Third, he arranges for Pook to wear a heart monitor for a month. The results from her thirty day trial are negative, with no episodes of AFIB.

We discuss whether he might consider her a candidate for a technique called ablation, which can eliminate AFIB episodes entirely. He indicates that she is not a good candidate because of the risks involved with such surgery at her age. Finally he recommends that Pook begin taking Warfarin/Coumadin as protection against a stroke, but leaves the decision up to me.

While she is laid up with a wheelchair and then a walker, I get my first real taste of becoming chief cook, grocer and kitchen cleaner. Fortunately, she is close enough by my side to coach me through recipes and needed food purchases.

CHAPTER 8 –ADDING A LEWY BODY DEMENTIA DIAGNOSIS

PD Doctor Visit and Communications

We have our six months appointment with her PD doctor on May 16. I provide him with the following summary of her current medical condition:

Surgery

She had hip replacement surgery on her right leg on March 8. The morning after surgery she had an episode of atrial fibrillation, followed by two more episodes within the next six or seven days.

She has now completed two weeks of outpatient therapy; continues with some therapy exercises at home; walks without a cane, but with some limping; walks up and down stairs in normal fashion (we have four stories in our condo), and is cleared to ride a bicycle

Medication

She had been taking one 25/100 Sinemet pill, three times per day, since last July; began taking 1-1/2 pills the first week in February, because of concern over feeling stiff in the morning, combined with her pre-surgery right leg pain problems; uncertain if the increased dosage helps.

She takes a multivitamin and calcium and vitamin D supplements each morning; takes one 81 mg aspirin each morning; one 25 mg Metropolol with breakfast and dinner for heart rate control.

Exercise

She and I have now resumed playing ping pong every other day. She plays well with great coordination, hitting the ball from both the forehand and backhand sides; both of us enjoying a lot of laughs over missed or badly struck balls. However, she still has difficulty bending down to pick balls up off the floor.

We take a short 10 to 15 minute walk every day and she began bicycling again yesterday, with an initial ten minute ride.

Sleep Problems

She has trouble sleeping every night; stays in bed typically from 11:00 PM or so till about 3:00 AM, then goes downstairs and sleeps on a family room *couch; stays there till about 9:00 AM before getting dressed. She periodically complains of restless legs at night.*

She mostly sleeps on her back with both legs bent at the knee. Her legs sometimes twitch while sleeping and she will sometimes open her mouth and emit one brief snore, waking her up.

Her doctor takes Pook through a bunch of mental tests such as:

> *Gives her three simple unrelated words like car, dog and chair, and tells her he's going to ask her to recall those words in five or ten minutes.*
> *Asks-Where is she; what floor she's on?*
> *What city are we in; what city does she live in?*
> *What county does she live in?*
> *Who is the President?*
> *What month is this and what day?*
> *Gives her a drawing of a three dimensional figure and asks her to copy it.*

She fails almost every question.

He then surprises us, adding an additional diagnosis - she has Lewy Body Dementia (LBD).

I have realized that she has shown some mental issues but discounted them as just being evidence of mild cognitive impairment. The word "dementia" is an immediate shocker and raises concerns about the future – is she going to quickly forget who I am; or the kids and grandkids? Her brother, who also had Parkinson's, went for about 8 years before any dementia showed up. The doctor, who we both like and respect, cannot forecast what the long-term prognosis might be for her, since, like PD, every patient reacts differently. He prescribes a drug called Aricept to possibly help her with LBD memory problems.

Pook is shook with this new diagnosis and begins sobbing as soon as we get back in the car. She continues with questions about what is going to happen to her, before falling asleep after about ten or fifteen minutes later, and remains asleep during the remainder of the drive home. We will continue to discuss LBD over the course of the next several days with her seemingly much less anxious once I assure her that she doesn't have Alzheimer's; that people with LBD usually have accompanying hallucinations, which she doesn't have; and that no specific test is available to prove that she really has LBD.

CHAPTER 9 – MY CAREGIVER ACTIONS

I look up Parkinson's dementia aspects; Aricept as related to PD; and Lewy Body Dementia, finding:

1. The relationship between PD and dementia is covered in an article I come across. Only 20% of people with PD will be expected to develop dementia (PDD). For those who go on to develop PDD, there is usually a 10-15 year lag time between Parkinson diagnosis and the onset of dementia.

2. The doctor's Aricept prescription comes as a huge shock – normally prescribed for Alzheimer's patients. I uncover several studies of the use of Aricept with patients having PDD or LBD. These studies demonstrate positive results for the patients in both cases, in terms of cognition and behavior, supporting the hypothesis that both diseases are closely related.

3. Lewy Body Dementia is characterized, in a Mayo Clinic article, as the second most common type of progressive dementia after Alzheimer's. It also may cause visual hallucinations, seeing shapes, colors, people or animals that aren't there, or even having

conversations with deceased loved ones. I recall that one day, following her PD diagnosis, Pook had yelled up to me: "Dad, is mom up there" - many, many years since her parents had passed away. In Lewy Body dementia, abnormal round structures, called Lewy bodies, develop in regions of your brain involved in thinking and movement. It causes confusion and memory loss; reduced attention span; frequent episodes of drowsiness; long periods of staring into space and disorganized speech. I have already noticed evidence of all these symptoms occurring with Pook.

4. LBD presents concerns not only about memory loss versus time, but also the question of average life expectancy. The Mayo Clinic report goes on to say that signs and symptoms will worsen with time, causing the dementia to get worse. Furthermore, death, on average, takes place about eight years after onset.

5. What should I now begin doing different with her as her caregiver? The Mayo article recommends: enhance communications by touching an arm or shoulder to focus attention; encourage exercise for improved strength and cardiovascular health, to retain motor skills and produce a calming effect; listen to calming music

My professional background includes a lot of work on various aspects of planning for the future. So I assemble a plan I call "Pook's Health Improvement Plan". My plan is an extensive shopping list of activities we can do together, and with others, that should help her retain her health despite both her progressive diseases – PD and LBD. Optimistically, and overly ambitious, I envision that all together we can devote some 4 or 5 hours per day to these activities.

Pook's Health Improvement Plan

1. Aerobic exercise: Fast walks, biking, ping pong, Nintendo WII TV dancing
2. Physical recreational exercise: Dumbbell workouts, yoga, Nintendo WII sports, golf practice and playing
3. Mental pursuits: Playing gin rummy, typing emails and letters, keyboard music practice, memorizing poetry, various social activities with friends, kids and grandkids

I will gradually reduce the lists over the next month or so as we try different ideas, but many of the items on the list will remain there, and be regularly pursued for the next several years. I am full of fear and depression, feeling we have entered a long dark tunnel with walls defined by the limits of her two major diseases; with huge concerns about her reduced life expectancy. What am I to tell the kids?

A brief touch of humor

The next night she takes her first Aricept pill, only one half of one to start. No side effects are apparent. I thought, or just hoped, that she was a bit more talkative the next morning. That day one of our grandkids, Nick, comes over to get my help for an artistic wood picture (Intarsia) he's working on. Pook makes us sandwiches and Nick's favorite blueberry muffins and complementing him on the wood work he has done thus far. That night our daughter Kari calls - laughing. When she came home from work, Nick immediately questioned her – "What happened to Grandma, did she just have some kind of surgery? Today she seemed like my same old Grandma – we sat at the table and talked, with her asking me a lot of questions". One day and one-half pill - is a miracle in store for us? Two days, from deep depression to hope!

PD/LBD doctor communication

I send an email to her doctor two weeks later to apprise him of the Aricept results thus far and raise some questions. My comments to him regarding her response to the Aricept are:

> *Her conversational ability has improved; she recalls each day's events better; she has improved in her meals preparation activity, planning and following recipes better; she still cannot recall three simple words after five minutes, like the way you tested her.*

I question him regarding whether some way exists to pinpoint the type of dementia she has, based on his research work regarding brain imaging techniques:

> *I am troubled by four questions regarding Pook's mental health, following up on your Aricept prescription for her:*
>
> 1. *What is the specific source of her apparent mild dementia?*
> 2. *What does that source imply regarding her prognosis?*

3. Should she be given some type of imaging test to attempt to isolate the specific source?
4. Would such imaging be of value to track her future progress?

Unfortunately, his answer comes back that no imaging technique yet exists to differentiate different kinds of dementia, except for Alzheimer's.

May/June/July Activities

Pook's memory difficulties, clearly pointed out with her LBD diagnosis, don't have any discernible impact on her day to day life and activities. Her personality remains essentially the same and she can do most everything she was already doing, as constrained by her PD. So the middle of the summer includes:

> She completes her therapy session, necessary following her hip replacement surgery in early May
>
> We golf by ourselves and she golfs with her girl-friends, still driving alone to the various golf courses where they usually play

We take long walks most days of the week; she shows none of the typical PD characteristics, such as shuffling along; her left arm doesn't swing as far as the right one, but not a noticeable difference

We bicycle over a four mile route through our neighborhood; also bike an 8 mile circuit through a nearby metro park

We watch sports activities of many of our 14 grandkids, especially soccer

We participate in two grandkids high school graduations and graduation parties

We drive to visit two western Michigan cities and have a great visit, touring shops and galleries as has become sort of a joint hobby over the years; buy ourselves a nice set of oil-fed candles for the dining room.

CHAPTER 10 – COMBINED AFIB AND LBD TREATMENTS – AND FUN

My Caregiver Actions

I read an article on the LBD Association web site which is headed by these words: "A comprehensive approach to treatment can significantly improve the quality of life of patients with Lewy Body Dementia". The body of the article goes on to say that LBD patients can improve with therapy, sometimes markedly, and do quite well, for many, many years. I vow to pursue therapy – both mental and physical – for Pook. I search the Web for mental exercise ideas and come up with the following four:

1. Memorizing poetry
2. Spelling practice – spelling words both forwards and backwards
3. Recalling word orders – viewing a list of words and then recalling their order of appearance
4. Solving word search puzzles

So I begin what I call "LBD School" with Pook, five days a week, starting around 4:00 PM and lasting thirty to forty minutes. The plan is for us to work together on one or more of these mental exercises each day. LBD School becomes one of the most rewarding caregiver ideas I will have – stimulating her brain; becoming a source of facial improvement exercises; and a source of lots of spontaneous laughter for the two of us.

1. **Memorizing poetry**

I search the Web for poetry verses that are humorous, and sufficiently brief to learn. I find the following poem which is perfect for our needs. (And which, amazingly, will still be retained in her mind almost four years later, even after she has had a major stroke!)

How to Paint a Wall

When I went off to work one day,
She decided to paint a wall,
When I came back home that night,
She was curled into a ball.

Her eyes were closed, she was breathing hard,
Her hair was very wet,
From her head to the tips of her pretty toes,
She was covered all in sweat.

She was wrapped in a jacket made of down,
With a fur coat on top of that,

The wall was glowing with new, fresh paint,
On the floor, the paint can sat.

"Sweetheart!" I cried, with a worried look,
"Are you all right my dear?"
She lazily opened her lovely eyes,
And smiled from ear to ear.

"I knew I could do it", she said with a grin;
"I followed the paint can notes,
It clearly said for best results,
Be sure to put on two coats."

By Joanna Fuchs

I decide to proceed with learning the poem together on a responsive basis – I would say the first line, she would say the second, I the third, and so on through the entire poem. I am pleasantly surprised with how well, and quickly, the memorization proceeds, even though neither of us has had occasion to learn any poetry since our days in high school. We learn the first verse in only about a week. As we work through memorizing the second verse and adding it to the second, this expected chore becomes the source of loads of laughter as we take turns in making recitation mistakes. Continuing along with adding other verses, we laugh more, longer and more intensely – sometimes hanging on to each other as we laugh, or our laughter being so strong it bring tears to our eyes. Our intended mental therapy work becomes a terrific source of everyday fun. All the laughter brings forth noticeable improvement in her facial expression abilities as we proceed over the weeks and months.

Within a short several months we can regularly recite what has become "our" poem and proudly demonstrate our achievement to our kids and grandkids when we get together – a huge positive surprise to our kids, who have been so concerned about her future with LBD, ever since hearing the doctor's formidable diagnosis of LBD.

Thrilled by our success on this first poem, I hunt for a second to work on. I recall a book of poetry that I used to read to our kids when they were small, called "The Golden Treasury of Poetry". One often read poem in particular comes to mind:

The Raggedy Man

Oh the Raggedy Man, he works for pa,
And he's the goodest man ever you saw,
He comes to our house every day,
And waters the horses and feeds them hay,
And opens our shed, and we all just laugh,
When he drives out our little old wobbely calf,
And then, if our hired girl says he can.
He milks the cow for 'Lizabeth Ann,
Ain't he an awful good Raggedy Man?

        Raggedy, Raggedy, Raggedy Man!

Why the Raggedy Man is so good,
He splits the kindling, and chops the wood,
And then he spades in our garden too,
And does most thing that boys can't do,
He climbed clean up in ur big tree,
And shooked down an apple for me,
And another one too for 'lizabeth Ann,
And another one too for the Raggedy Man,
Ain't he an awful kind Raggedy Man?
        Raggedy, Raggedy, Raggedy Man!

And the Raggedy Man, knows most Rhymes,
And tells them, if I be good sometimes,
Knows about Giants and Griffons and Elves,
And the Squidgicum Squees that swallers themselves,
And right by the pump in our pasture lot,
He showed me the hole that the Wunks has got,
That lives way down deep in the ground, and can,
Turn into me or 'Lizabeth Ann,
Or Ma or Pa or the Raggedy Man,
Ain't he a funny Raggedy Man?
        Raggedy, Raggedy, Raggedy Man!

The Raggedy Man, one time when he,
 Was making a little bow and arrow for me,
Says, "When you are big like your Pa is,
Ain't you going to have a fine store like his,
And be a rich merchant, and wear fine clothes,

And what are you going to be, goodness knows"!
And then he laughed at 'Lizabeth Ann,
And I says, "I'm just going to be a Raggedy Man,
I'm just going to be a nice Raggedy Man,
      Raggedy, Raggedy, Raggedy Man!

James Whitcomb Riley

This poem of four long, ten line verses, with a built-in accent, appears much tougher to learn, but it has the advantage of familiarity from the "good old days" of reading it over and over to our then children. We forge ahead remarkably fast and can recite it with only occasional small errors by Christmas.

2. Spelling Practice

Our one daughter has four dyslexic sons. From time to time I have tutored each of them on reading and spelling. During this tutoring period I have acquired a supportive "kit" which includes a series of four by six spiral bound cards. Each card contains a single word in large print. The set of spiral bound words is graded by difficulty. I select several of these cards to use in Pook's spelling sessions, and start with simple four letter words with simple syllables like "rope, jeep, and pill". I hold a word up in front of her, ask her to say the word, then give her about 10 seconds to look at it in order to be able to visualize it. I take the card away and ask her "say the word"; then "spell the word"; then "spell the word backwards". If she has trouble remembering the word, I'll show it to her again, a little longer the second time. It takes several weeks of practice before she becomes comfortable with the process, and with being able to hold a word in her memory long enough to spell it backwards.

She gradually advances to longer and more difficult multi-syllable words, such as "ocean, purple, and lotion". I introduce words with double vowels and consonants such as "clapped, raffle, and crooked". I'm amazed that, having been diagnosed with LBD, she is able to master spelling such difficult words backwards. Each session lasts 20 or 30 minutes, depending on how well she does or how tired she seems to be. She will get anywhere from 50 to 75% of the spellings correct in both directions on her first try on a good day. Just like when she is memorizing poetry, she will sometimes catch herself making a mistake and start laughing out loud, with me joining in. With this light hearted tone for our work, she seems happy to begin whenever I suggest that it's time for spelling class.

3. Learning columns of words

I type up lists of words one above another in straight columns, beginning with short four letter words, lined up into a column of only four words. The idea is for her to look at the column of words for 15 to 30 seconds, close her eyes and be able to say them back to me in order - both top to bottom and bottom to top. I gradually proceed to longer words and longer columns of words. This turns out to be a very difficult exercise for her. Over the course of maybe a month, we work up to a six word column, containing six letter words. She struggles and struggles to recall the order. Then I complicate the exercise by asking her to recall just the first or last three words; then the first and last word. She finds it difficult, makes a lot of mistakes as I vary the sequences she's asked for, but she keeps trying and we laugh a lot, maybe only doing one or two six word sets in half an hour.

4. Word Search

In the past, before any of her health problems, she would sometimes enjoy doing the newspaper's "word search" puzzle, as I did the crossword puzzle. The word search problem is laid out on a page as a grid of maybe 20 letters by 20 letters, seemingly in random order. A list of words to be located within the puzzle is usually provided along-side, or directly under, the puzzle. Usually the words to be found are all part of some defined category, such as "names of careers". The challenge is to find each of the listed words, which might be located vertically, sideways or diagonally within the grid of 400 letters. I buy a book containing only word search puzzles, and some days she will sit alone on the sofa and relax, doing one page of the word search book. I don't attempt to assist her in any way, but she will proudly show me her successful completions. She obviously takes pleasure in concentrating on such puzzles. She's slow, and each puzzle takes her two to three hours, but, for now, continues doing them.

Physical Exercises

Our normal outdoor activities continue into August. One day, as we are bike riding around our small lake on individual bikes, she jerks as a car passes us without warning and seemingly too close, running her into an adjacent curb and falling on her bike. She just gets a small bleeding scratch on her leg, but it scares her and she decides to give up bike riding. A few weeks later we go to our nearby metro par, where we have been bike riding for years. She reads a book while I ride. I miss her usual company on my ride, and only do this once or twice more before giving up on riding there as a single.

As winter approaches, we need to resume one or more indoor exercise programs. I locate a Tai Chi class and we visit as observers, but feel it's too far to drive weekly. We also tour a hospital related exercise facility but feel they don't offer enough classes outside of just using the equipment. We then watch yoga and water aerobics sessions at the local health club where we used to play tennis. We sign up for both classes; one hour of yoga once a week; and one hour of water aerobics twice a week. She doesn't like the yoga after two sessions so we instead join a weekly one hour session for seniors only, called "strength and stretch". The class includes the use of equipment such as dumbbells, stretch ropes and inflated balls, allowing each participant to select the pieces of equipment that best suits their needs and strength.

As the weather turns colder we resume mall walking once or twice a week and play ping pong in our basement in addition to our sports club exercises program.

CHAPTER 11 – NOVEMBER DOCTOR VISITS

1. AFIB Doctor

My update note to her doctor:

Current Medications

>*Takes one 25 MG Metoprolol each with breakfast and dinner*
>
>*Takes one 325 MG aspirin each evening before going to bed (except when taking a sleeping pill, not wishing to mix the two).*
>
>*Takes 1-1/2 pills of 10 MG Donepezil (Aricept) each morning*
>
>*Takes 25/100 Sinemet at 8:00 AM; 2:00 PM; and 8:00 PM each da*
>
>*Takes Caltrate plus D vitamin plus a multi-vitamin each morning*

Exercise Program

>*Began sports club exercising in mid-September; nominally does one hour of water aerobics twice*

per week; one hour of senior strength and stretch each week. One hour of Yoga proved to be too much; planning to begin one or two 20 minute Yoga sessions each week at home in the near future

Has been walking about one mile about three times per week, weather permitting; will change to mall walking (one mile) as weather gets colder.

Personal health

Parkinson's has worsened in terms of right hand tremors, both at rest and when eating. Other symptoms to be evaluated by her PD doctor tomorrow

Lewy Body Dementia is also apparently worse in terms of personality impact and memory loss

She no longer drives

Still shares the cooking; washes dishes; washes clothes; vacuums; makes beds, etc
.
Dresses herself and puts on/removes make-up every day

Current Situation and Concerns

Husband takes her blood pressure and pulse each morning and evening. Occasionally checks BP and pulse after exercising, with no AFIB problems having occurred.

She continues to have infrequent AFIB episodes, with her heart rate at less than 100-105 BPM; I give her an additional 25 MG Metroprolol pill and she recovers usually within eight hours.

I prefer not to place her on Coumadin because of: the extra complexity involved in her already complex treatments; concerns about Coumadin side effects; feel she is a low-risk patient with no evidence of ischemic attacks or other heart problems and no high cholesterol. The benefits of Coumadin over Aspirin do not appear that significant. Her other health problems, especially Lewy Body Dementia, are of much greater concern.

We have a brief meeting with her doctor feeling that she's doing fine with current medication; sets a follow-up meeting with his nurse practitioner for six months later.

2. PD/LBD Doctor Visit

I present him with the following note:

1. <u>Her status re Parkinson's</u>

    She is now experiencing essential tremors in her right hand, and sometimes in her right leg, in addition to her Parkinson's based tremors. These essential tremors are bad enough that they interfere with her eating – she has had to switch to using her left hand when drinking coffee or tea; now uses the fork in her left hand with dinner, and a spoon in her left hand when eating breakfast cereal.

    She has begun experiencing a repetitive chewing motion with her tongue and lips, leading to a somewhat "sneering" look on her face at times. She recognizes that this is happening but has no control over it.

    She has been walking just fine and swinging her arms nicely, going about one mile during good weather days, (through October) though I have to keep reminding her to keep her head up and looking around(otherwise tends to look at the sidewalk about 10 or 15 feet ahead of her, almost like she's hypnotized). She also leans slightly forward.

She biked about 3-1/2 miles with me two or three times per week through August.

She began health club exercises in September - water aerobics for one hour, two times per week; senior strength and stretch for one hour, once per week. Hope to resume limited Yoga at home for ½ hour once or twice per week; plus ½ hour morning mall walking twice per week, depending on how well she sleeps.

2. <u>Her status re Lewy Body Dementia</u>

I am mostly concerned about her dementia which seems to be rapidly getting worse. I increased her dosage of Aricept from 5 mg to 10 mg to 15 mg but no longer see it helping her memory.

She does really well in mental exercises which we do regularly each day and have fun while doing them.

She used to be very conversational, but can no longer hold a conversation with people anymore; does not volunteer sentences in a small group discussion; when asked a direct question just answers with one brief sentence. She knows that her mind is slow, making her unable to participate, and is highly bothered.

> *She has had several episodes of mental confusion when in unfamiliar places, such as ladies locker room at water aerobics*
>
> *She no longer drives due to a dangerous confusion incident (ignoring a red traffic light)*
>
> *She can no longer handle banking details that she has taken care of for years*
>
> *She still does routine things like washing clothes and dishes; cooking (we sometimes split the work, although I'm taking over more and more); vacuuming; and still applies her makeup (left-handed) each morning and removes it each night. No problems dressing or undressing or taking showers*

Sleep - She sleeps poorly at night. Goes to bed about 10:30 to 11:00 PM; gets up twice or so during the night. Often wakes up about 3:00 or 4:00 AM, complaining she can't sleep; goes down stairs and tries to fall asleep on the sofa with mixed results. Complains of lack of sleep and being tired each morning. Sleeping pill doesn't seem to help.

Question 1: Her fast onset of dementia is my biggest worry – if she continues the recent trend, how bad might she become in just the next year? She recognizes that she has lost so much memory and worries about it. Can you suggest any type of additional treatment that might help her memory?

Question 2: Her AFIB doctor has recommended she take Coumadin for stroke prevention. I have read that it raises the possibility of "causing cognitive malfunction". Any studies that support that possibility?

Note to Family Regarding Mom's Health

We met yesterday with her heart doctor; and today with her Parkinson's doctor. Both appointments went better than expected.

AFIB doctor visit

> I provided him with a 1-1/2 page summary of her AFIB episodes during the past five months and he seemed quite bored with the entire meeting. Yes, we're doing the right things monitoring her blood pressure and pulse every day; watching for her AFIB and giving her an extra half pill each time she has an episode, which usually takes her about 4 or 5 hours to recover. He feels that to have four or five such episodes each month isn't a big deal.
>
> Her next appointment isn't until next June and then just with his nurse practitioner

PD/LBD doctor visit

> I also wrote up a 1-1/2 summary for him which he reviewed; then checked her physically. He was pleasantly surprised at how well she's doing; what good physical condition she's in. He basically feels that she hasn't deteriorated at all physically over

the past two years he has been seeing her and feels that this is remarkable compared to the usual patient he sees. He doesn't feel that her increasing right hand tremors are that unusual and no added medication is required. He's also pleased that her PD hasn't crossed over to her left side thus far.

His mental checks indicate that she hasn't changed at all from the last and previous visits and shouldn't be expected to deteriorate any more over the next two years

He was especially surprised, and smiled broadly, at her ability to memorize her part of a five verse poem, and felt that such exercises should continue as part of her treatment. He went on to explain that she does not have Alzheimer's; that with Lewy Body Dementia her functions have just slowed down and aren't disappearing, the reason for her difficulty in conversations. He recommended further work with relatively simple jigsaw puzzles and other games, such as UNO, to keep her interested in mental work.

We discussed her sleep problems and he feels that it's probably just a perception and that she sleeps more than she realizes. She can continue to take over the counter sleep medications, such as Simply Sleep, if she feels she's getting benefit, but doesn't want to prescribe a sleep med, which he doesn't feel is necessary and could do some harm.

CHAPTER 12 – HER HEALTH IMPACTS

As we entered 2011 we had already learned to live with Pook having PD, and adapted our lifestyle accordingly – the most noticeable difference being having to give up tennis due to her PD imposed slowness and loss of coordination. She could still walk just fine, swinging her arms reasonably well and going for one to two mile walks; still rode a bike and still played golf, driving her-self to golf with lady friends. Tremors were a big nuisance but didn't hamper her daily life that much.

But the year 2011 brought with it new surprises, requiring additional medication and lifestyle adaptation. First came the shock of AFIB, followed only two months later by the diagnosis of an added progressive disease – Lewy Body Dementia. AFIB adaptation required a change of doctors; more medication to track; daily checks of Pook's pulse; and a choice between daily use of Coumadin or Aspirin for stroke prevention.

The advent of LBD has marked a major near term intrusion on Pook's world, particularly the loss of her freedom to drive herself whenever and wherever she wanted to go;

has also impacted her thought process, removing her abilities to write checks, balance a checkbook and handle banking transactions. She can still, however, dress herself, put on and take off makeup and perform many household chores that she is used to doing.

The LBD diagnosis was immediately depressing because of the implications for her long-term future – when might dementia take away her ability to know all the people – kids, grandkids and friends she has been so close to.

However I will forever remember the uplift we have received from all the good days working together on mental exercises – amazed at how well she has done; the remarkable result in fun and laughter; the return of much of her personality; the pleasure of seeing emotions returning on her face; how we received similar benefits from our two short road trips to upper Michigan. Those brief trips brought us back to our usual avocation of touring through small shops; buying some items for the house; visiting some Michigan wineries, and purchasing a few bottles of their different wines; searching out unusual eating places; and buying her one delightful, unusual jacket to wear; with tremors only rarely bothersome. The capabilities she lost through PD and LBD were mostly forgotten with the several months of fun together.

CHAPTER 13 – CAREGIVER LESSONS LEARNED

The year 2011 reinforced a number of caregiver lessons that began last year:

>The importance of doctor communications and doctor selection

>The necessity of delving into medical based articles on the Internet, full of complicated terms, expanding my vocabulary. This has only gotten more complicated.

>The need to understand Pook's needs and follow-up on actions to help her cope with the restrictions of her changing health picture. This again has only gotten more difficult.

>The need to emphasize our continuing happiness through creative ways to have fun, while avoiding dwelling on negative and depressing aspects of her, thus far, downward health journey.

2011 has also brought forth additional responsibilities:

The increasing recognition that I'm not just a caregiver in the sense of keeping her comfortable, but that I'm also a "disease fighter". The doctors supply the pills that help control her symptoms, and provide advice, such as "spend a lot of time on exercise", that's more important than the pills". So I'm responsible for taking actions that will improve her long-term health outlook, such as enrolling her in specific types of exercise classes, and actions defining specific approaches to mental exercises to keep her brain alert.

With regard to the "disease fighter" responsibility, I must have daily discipline – that for her well-being I must follow schedules to ensure that she is daily spending sufficient time on mental and physical exercise, both at home and at wherever we find outside help.

Being able to handle the complexities of multi-tasking – taking over paying bills and banking; participating in grocery shopping and, increasingly, cooking; in addition to the disease fighting tasks, handing out pills, getting to doctor appointments, communicating with them and others. Increasingly, there seems to be insufficient time to do everything as well as you feel you should.

Searching for enjoyment activities beyond looking to keep her comfortable and disease fighting.

YEAR 2012 – COPING WITH PD/LBD HEALTH COMPLEXITY

CHAPTER 14 – EXTENDING 2011 KNOWLEDGE AND CAPABILITIES

At the beginning of year 2011, Pook and I were both concerned about her Parkinson's disease symptoms – especially slowness of movement, mask face, and tremors; and what was the best response to enable her to enjoy life despite PD limitations. Together we mourned her loss of tennis playing, after thirty or more years or so of such good exercise and enjoyment. PD medication had begun to assist with facial symptoms and she was coping with tremors reasonably well. Then the diagnosis of AFIB and LBD came along as new health shocks. By the end of 2011 we had found a PD doctor that we liked and had confidence in; understood the nature of her AFIB and she had begun taking medication to limit its impacts. We had also begun a program to minimize and/or slow down the impacts of LBD, through a combination of mental and physical exercises. The mental exercise program had already shown benefits, uncovering new chances for working and laughing together.

So we entered our 57th year of marriage together with our spirits excellent, despite two progressive diseases intruding into her health. We looked forward to enjoyable daily physical and mental exercise programs to maintain her near-term health during 2012. Since she had become too nervous to bike by herself any longer, I ordered a tandem bike in January. Since it would be coming from China, it wouldn't be delivered until sometime in April. We still expected the possibility of a cruise to some place in the Caribbean; a winter trip to visit her sister in Arizona, as well some shorter trips within Michigan, like we had done in the latter part of 2011; and maybe even a longer drive back to our home state of North Dakota.

My Caregiver Goals and Actions

I establish an early personal goal for this year: <u>Explore the Web further for research on symptoms improvements, and potential cures, for PD and LBD</u>. Some of my initial finds:

> An LBD study site is studying caregiver's and their roles. It is conducting a survey which takes only 30 minutes and I respond; but never get the overall survey results.

A startling press release from Case Western Reserve School of Medicine, referencing an article just being published in Science magazine, states: "I am pleased to report that our neuroscience faculty have made a dramatic breakthrough in the battle against Alzheimer's disease. Tomorrow's edition of the Journal of Science will report on how Professor Gary Landreth and his team discovered that a cancer drug can quickly reverse Alzheimer's symptoms in animal models. Within 72 hours of administration, this medication halved the number of plaque deposits closely associated with this degenerative brain disease. More, it saw the signs of cognitive and memory deficits disappear within the same short time period". The world is agog with this news and immediately AD patients and caregivers are clamoring for samples of this medicine – Bexarotene - to try out. Unfortunately, as the world soon finds that such a "quick fix" does not prove to be the eagerly anticipated solution for AD and other forms of dementia.

More in my direct interest is a study of the use of Donepezil for LBD patients, which indicates benefits in a majority of patients, as I have already experienced with Pook.

Actions

I take direct action toward improving Pook's exercise options and coordination by purchasing Nintendo WII materials – WII Sports and WII Sports Resort CD's. These CD's allow us to go through the motions of swinging a baseball bat, a tennis racket, golf club or bowling ball, by using the appropriate motions, while waving a wand at a sensor mounted atop the TV. We try the various sports by ourselves and with family members. We have some good laughs during these trials but, unfortunately, Pook just can't swing the wand with needed timing, and is also hampered by tremors as she tries to use her right hand, so we give up on the possibility of her personal participation.

Pook's health altering accidents

In early January, Pook faints or trips on a mat in the kitchen, while emptying the dishwasher, falls and breaks her ankle. The doctor places her in a walking boot for four to six weeks while it's healing. The walking boot is quite awkward so she limps around the house doing normal housework.

In late January Pook faints in the bathroom while doing her hair, falls against the toilet and breaks it. I bring a bar stool up from our basement and luckily find that it fits perfectly in an open space between the "his and her" sinks. While doing her hair or makeup in the future I intend to make sure that she's always seated.

A week later, while I'm upstairs, she doesn't realize where I am and goes out the front door, without me hearing the door open and close. She heads for our usual walking path through the adjacent woods, searching for me, even though hobbled by the walking boot. A while later I come downstairs and immediately notice that she's gone, with no idea where she might have went. I look a block or so away, by our community mailbox, in case she had just walked out to mail a letter, but she isn't around there. I return home to decide where to look next and see her just turning onto the sidewalk entrance to our condo; run out in time to catch her as she's about to collapse. This incident generates a new fear of leaving her alone because of the possibility of similar mental breakdowns.

Pook becomes nervous about the walking incident, and understands that she had a mental lapse. She begins to have increased tremors and AFIB episodes. She also has trouble sleeping, waking up in the middle of the night with severe tremors. I send the following fax to her PD doctor:

CHAPTER 15 – PD DOCTOR COMMUNICATIONS

My wife is the worst I've seen her - experiencing unusually lengthy and severe tremors in her right hand, causing anxiety, which has then triggered two atrial fibrillation episodes - Tuesday and Wednesday, with Wednesday's continuing into this morning. Would a temporary prescription of a tranquilizer, for maybe several weeks, be appropriate to assist in calming her down? Other possible approaches?

We have been looking forward, for two months, to visiting her sister in Arizona for a week, departing Tuesday, February 21. Because of this anxiety/AFIB link, I now feel we should cancel those trip plans.

Background

> *Mary fainted with low blood pressure – 70/38 - taken immediately after the episode, and broke her ankle on January 12. She was placed in a walking boot to heal; doctors' x-ray indicated her ankle was healed and the boot was removed Monday, February 13.*

She was forced to discontinue her daily and weekly exercise program while wearing the walking boot, leading to increased anxiety.

Tuesday, she woke up feeling anxious and was in AFIB when I checked her pulse at 8:00 AM. I gave her one 50 MG Metropolol and the episode lasted till 3:00 PM in the afternoon. Her right hand tremors were also bothering her all day, both at rest and when eating; she had difficulty trying to relax. I feel her tremors have gradually been getting worse ever since her loss of the exercise program.

Wednesday the resting tremors continued all day. At dinner time the tremors were so bad she could not cut her food and splashed orange juice all over trying to drink using her right hand. I stroked her forearm to help that hand relax, while she ate and drank with her left hand. After dinner we watched some TV for an hour or so; she went to the bathroom and came out walking slowly while shaking all over. I helped her to a sofa and proceeded to calm her down by again stroking her right arm. When I checked her vitals she was had a BP of 112/66 and pulse at 133 beats per minute. I gave her an extra Metropolol pill before she went to bed. At 8:30 AM this morning, her BP was 90/48; pulse 101, both coming down. She slept intermittently today, and remains very tense;

> *relaxes her right hand from tremors only if I stroke it for five or ten minutes.*
>
> *I wanted to resume her weekly exercise program this week but she is too anxious about the tremors to consider trying, even if not in AFIB.*

His nurse responds the next day, increasing her PD dosage from 1-1/2 pills to 2 pills, still three times a day. She also phones in a prescription to our drugstore for a tranquilizer.

Tuesday, February 21, 2012

I send her doctor this follow-up fax:

<u>Friday night, Feb. 17</u>

I gave her the two Sinemet you recommended at 8:00 PM Friday evening and she was fine watching a Red Wings game – no tremors. Went to bed about 11:15 PM.

<u>Saturday, February 18</u>

She woke me at 3:00 AM with bad tremors. I gave her a generic sleeping pill and massaged her forearm and hand for about an hour to ease the tremors till she fell asleep. She got up at 5:00 AM and slept till 8:00 AM; BP at 99/43; pulse 90, in AFIB, but no tremors. Gave her the two Sinemet and a 50 mg Metoprolol. She was in AFIB all day; had bad tremors off and on and when she walked to the bathroom shook all over bad that I had to escort her holding her arm. Went to bed at 11:15 PM; BP 94/51, pulse still 90.

Sunday, February 19

Woke up at 7:45 AM with pulse and tremors okay. Gave her two Sinemet at 8:00 AM. Seemed okay all day, but slept most of the day. Went to daughter's for dinner and no tremors; no AFIB.

Monday, February 20

Checked BP and pulse upon waking at 6:45 AM; both were fine; checked again at 9:45 AM because she was going to wash clothes and both still fine. Had some tremors at lunch, but not bad and slept some. Worked on a puzzle from about 3:00 PM to 3:45 PM and seemed fine, no tremors. Went for walk about 4:30 PM and had to turn around as she was feeling shaky. Bad tremors and AFIB continued overnight.

Tuesday, February 21

Woke at 6:15 AM. No tremors but still in AFIB. Gave her 50 mg Metoprolol and AFIB continued overnight. Gave her regular Sinemet doses.

Summary Perspective

1. She began experiencing AFIB and the bad tremors Tuesday, February 14, after having the boot for her broken ankle removed; this has continued almost every day since. I personally feel that both the tremors and AFIB are due to her lack of exercise since she broke her ankle on January 12. The problem now is to be able to resume her previous exercise program, which went so well, without triggering AFIB. I also feel that she has gone downhill mentally with her loss of exercise.

2. I have picked up your Buspirone 5 mg prescription for anxiety but have not given her any as yet. I'm hopeful that beginning to take it will relieve any anxiety about resuming exercise, keep her out of AFIB, and allow exercise resumption.

3. She has commented already about feeling "over-medicated". I have quit giving her Aricept while she is having these AFIB/tremors bouts to relieve her of some medication. If she begins taking Buspirone, should she try going back to just 1-1/2 Sinemet pills?

4. If she is having tremors when I give her the two Sinemet, it seems to take one hour for the Sinemet to kick in; then Sinemet wears off in three or four hours and tremors resume.

I'm still unsure about how much the AFIB and tremors relate to each other

PD/LBD Doctor Response

The doctor recommends that I resume some light exercise and continue giving her both the two Sinemet pills and the normal dosage Aricept, which she had been taking for her

LBD; but he doesn't want to try using the Buspirone at this time for anxiety. We go for several slow, light mall walks, sitting down for a while half-way through; also do some yoga exercises and some work with light dumb-bells down the basement. Over two days the tremors go way down and the AFIB episodes stop.

Pook's health improvement in March

I provided the following a summary status report to her brother's widow, highlighting Pook's improving health, on March 22.

The past two weeks have been really good ones for Mary Ellen:

> *No Atrial Fibrillation episodes*
>
> *Lots of good exercise programs – two hours each week of water aerobics, on Tuesdays and Thursdays at our sports club; plus one hour of what's called "strength and stretch" on Wednesdays*
>
> *Thirty to forty minutes of walking on other days – sometimes through the woods by us, when it's nice; sometimes down the street; sometimes walking through the mall. Her pace is good, her stride is good and she swings her arms well. She doesn't*

look like she has Parkinson's at all when she's walking.

She seems to have resting tremors very seldom. Instead she gets essential tremors when she does things. But we've found that for several hours after she exercises, even if it's just lifting some 5 pound dumb-bells, she doesn't have those tremors when she sits down to eat.

If just resting, she has a tendency to roll her tongue around inside her mouth; but when concentrating on reading that doesn't happen at all.

We work on memorizing poetry every day. She easily remembers a five verse poem we memorized over six months ago, which surprised her doctor back then. Now we're about half way through memorizing a longer poem, with four long, ten line verses.

We also practice spelling most every day – spelling words frontwards and <u>backwards!</u> It's amazing how well she does this on most days, extending her abilities all the way to some long words like "trained" or "trapped".

Writing remains a big problem, maybe because she doesn't have any occasions to write anything and I've begun paying the bills and balancing the checkbook. So I have begun working with her on writing words and sentences by hand.

And my cooking is getting better – last night we had curried shrimp with rice and condiments – coconut, raisins and mandarin orange slices. Come by sometime for a gourmet meal! 'Course she makes lunch most days, usually sandwiches on the George Forman, and we take turns doing dishes. She's also very fastidious about keeping the family room rug, plus Living room and dining room carpets, vacuumed every week.

CHAPTER 16 – CAREGIVING GETS MORE COMPLEX

I add a new goal: <u>Try to get her to communicate via hand written letters.</u> I continue with our regular work on poetry and spelling exercises.

> I take her blood pressure and pulse every morning to make sure her blood pressure isn't too low and that her pulse remains below 70, to make sure she isn't in AFIB. I worry if her blood pressure is too low, which I define as below 45, and if her heart is in AFIB with her heart rate much greater than 75 or 80. If her blood pressure is too low I'll walk her around slow and easy, and then check it again. When in AFIB, her heart rate usually doesn't go much above 100, and I will then give her an added one-half pill of Metropolol to reduce it. She tends to come out of AFIB within eight hours if I'm careful getting her to lie down and relax.
>
> I had her work on a poem "The Raggedy Man", beginning in January, which we both enjoy. We had learned it by some time into April. I searched for

another poem to work on and settled on "A Visit from St. Nicholas". Our pace is such that we are able to memorize about four lines or so every two weeks. Memorization gets tougher, of course, as we get further along, with more lines completed.

I begin working with her to hand write sentences, beginning by writing down sentences about subjects I pick out, such as today's weather. But I don't dictate any sentences, she has to pick out words and do her own spelling. As an example, when we got our new tandem bike I suggested that she write something about that. She writes "I got tandem bike yestore day".

She is gradually getting more comfortable doing this, until I am able to get her to write several sentences in a row. In June and July she writes several letters to her sister, my sister, her brother's widow and to our eldest son, with me encouraging her about what to say. She seems proud of each letter and I have begun keeping copies when we mail them out.

PD Doctor Visit and Communications

I write the following note to her PD/LBD doctor and present it to him at our regular six months meeting on May 29.

Current Exercise Programs, joint with husband

> *One hour of formal group water aerobics every Tuesday and Thursday morning*
>
> *One hour of a formal group "strength and stretch" program every Wednesday morning*
>
> *Tandem bike riding, four miles, three to five times per week, depending on weather; enjoys ride and pedaling along with freedom from gears shifting and balance worries*
>
> *Walks of 20-25 minutes several times per week, depending on weather; pace and stride are good along with swinging arms; shoulders sag forward and she tends to drop chin and eyes downward, needing reminders to keep head up.*
>
> *"Mental gymnastics", usually 30 to 45 minutes, four or five afternoons per week:*

Memorizing and reviewing poetry – knows two poems; working on a third

Spells words forward and backward, five to seven letters (examples – ocean; clapped)

Writes several dictated sentences; writes one sentence from her own thoughts

Memo: tired of doing word searches; tried working on brief (300 pieces) puzzle and could not select or fit pieces; no longer wants to play card games, like gin rummy

<u>Current Health Status</u>

Goes to bed each night about 11:00-11:30 PM

Wakes anywhere between 3:00 AM and 6:00 AM every morning with bad hand tremors; goes downstairs and lies on sofa; may or may not sleep further. Wakes again at about 7:00 AM, watches news and has decaf tea and a slice of toast; takes Sinemet and Metoprol pills. Usually has resting tremors watching news; essential tremors when eating breakfast cereal.

Reads books a lot during the day, seldom with noticeable resting tremors; otherwise spends a lot of time lying on sofa and staring ahead; cannot explain any thoughts except to say she's thinking about her health.

Has begun "tongue rolling" when not busy; face sometimes deteriorates into a "sneering" appearance. Neither apparent when concentrating on reading a book or when doing physical or mental exercises

No essential tremors for several hours after exercise.

No AFIB past 18 days; six months average of three AFIB episodes per month. AFIB is usually controlled with one additional Metoprolol pill; back to normal in four to six hours.

Feels shaky and has fainted once per month during the past six months – always due to her diastolic pressure falling below 45. Careful to have her sit down while putting on makeup because of uncertainty.

Current Functional Level

She still personally dresses herself; ties and double knots shoes; puts on and removes make-up and combs hair; remains concerned about appearance

Makes lunch about ½ of time. I make all dinners as she seems to no longer able to organize ingredients and follow recipes. She sets table; participates in making salads; helps doing dishes or does dishes alone sometimes.

She washes and dries clothes; vacuums; dusts

No trouble remembering names of four kids and spouses, 14 grandkids; address, phone number and garage door code. Sometimes recalls movie star names faster than I when watching a movie.

Struggles to remember yesterday's activities; sometimes forgets items mentioned maybe just one hour previous. Enjoys going to graduations, graduation dinners and parties.

Family Communications

Today we had Mary Ellen's six month checkup meeting with her PD/LBD Doctor at the University of Michigan. He took her through some physical and mental checks with the result that he's very pleased with her performance as he detects no substantial deterioration in either respect over the past year. He was especially surprised that she continues to walk at a good pace, with a good long stride, and does not have any signs of the typical Parkinson's shuffling gait. She also retains good flexibility in her hands, arms and feet. He re-emphasized how important exercise is to maintain her health; much more important than the pills she's taking; and liked the use of tandem biking. He's also pleased that she can memorize poetry and hold words in her mind long enough to spell them backwards.

He indicated that he is still uncertain whether she has Parkinson's disease, with some Lewy Body Disease characteristics added; or whether she basically has Lewy Body Disease, with some Parkinson's symptoms added. The difference could be important with respect to her long-term medication approach. The only way to tell for sure is through a new brain imaging technique the U of M researchers have developed that is some variation of MRI scanning. He went ahead and recommended her for testing under their current research program. If she fits their criteria for inclusion we should get a call from them in the next week or so.

I mentioned that she wakes up most nights at three or four in the morning with severe tremors in her right hand and arm, and those tremors continue till after she has had her morning dose of Sinemet with breakfast. They now have an extended release form of Sinemet and he gave her a prescription to take a minimal one-half pill dose each night at bedtime to see if that won't keep her from experiencing the tremors in the wee hours and allow her to sleep better.

This extended release pill is exactly what Pook needs, and she resumes sleeping normal hours. We don't see him again until November.

CHAPTER 17 – SUMMER ACTIVITIES

I pick up our new tandem bike near the end of April, just in time for the return of nice enough weather to use it several days a week. It's an instantaneous hit with twenty gears to assist our pedaling over the reasonable slopes around our neighborhoods. She just has to pedal and not worry about what gear to shift into. With me in front and doing the steering, she is also confident about our balance and direction. We soon become a frequent neighborhood sight and are greeted by waves and comments. On the nicest days she wants to go twice. One evening we are invited to our daughter's for dinner with her family, so we bike the two and one-half miles over, surprising everyone.

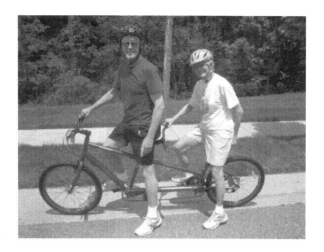

We continue with strength and stretch exercises, only doing them ourselves in our basement, but keep up water aerobics at our health club, with water aerobics now moving to an outside swimming pool. We also go for twenty to thirty minute walks through our nearby woods when it's too hot for bike rides.

I also want to keep up our travels, which have been such a nice part of our married lives through the years, and, I feel, are good therapy for her to get away from the same home bound routine. So I plan another one day trip to the city of Saugatuck, Michigan. This turns out to be too much of a departure for her. She sleeps a lot in the car, but is obviously nervous when we begin our usual tour of Saugatuck shops, asking a number of times - "Where are we going"? After we park and begin to stroll along the streets, she is insecure and wants to hold my hand or arm all the time. Our first visit is to a gift shop, one where we have previously bought some oil candles for our home. She helps me pick out a candle set for my sister and brother-in-law's anniversary but, as we exit, won't go further down that street. As we pass the kind of unusual shops we normally love to browse around in, she refuses to even enter. We walk only about two blocks and she insists that her legs hurt. We stop for lunch and she keeps asking "When are we going home?" She appears to be near tears. So we stay in the city less than two hours before heading back home.

Pook is recommended as a participant in a U of M research study whose purpose is testing a new PD sensing approach. I discuss what the study might mean for her and what she'll be doing during the related tests. I tell her I think her participation is a good idea, she agrees and we accept. The nature and purpose of the study is as follows:

"This project involves brain imaging with positron emission tomography (PET) and magnetic resonance imaging (MRI) in patient subjects with neurodegenerative diseases. Neurodegenerative diseases such as Alzheimer's disease (AD) and Parkinson's disease (PD), as well as a number of related cognitive and movement disorders, are increasingly prevalent in our aging population and there are no curative treatments currently available. A particular chemical in the brain, acetylcholine, is thought to play a key role in the development of these diseases. Methods to assess this chemical in the living brain are therefore crucial in the understanding of these diseases and in promoting the development of novel treatments. The primary purpose of this study is to test if brain "pictures" made with a new radiotracer, F-FEOBV, can provide satisfactory measures of acetylcholine activity in the brains of human subjects".

The description of study activities goes on to explain that the study will involve two phases: (1) eligibility and screening studies; and (2) the actual PET brain scanning.

CHAPTER 18 – PARKINSON'S ONLINE COURSE

In August I learn about a PD online course provided by the Parkinson's Foundation (PDF). The title of the course is "Parkinson's Advocates in Research Online Course". PDF's purpose in offering the course is to encourage community involvement in research, by providing individuals with scientific knowledge and leadership skills needed to take research to the next level. Upon completion of the course, an individual will be qualified to work as one of PDF's 180 Research Advocates. The course consists of four parts, each which is expected to take one hour to complete. Having a professional background in market and product planning, and having done a lot of personal PD research on the web, I am immediately intrigued. I would like very much to be able to participate in some type of communications with research personnel, providing practical insights based on my experiences with Pook.

I sign up for the course and, over a period of several weeks in August and September, complete the necessary four sections, answering test questions after each completion.

1. Clinical Research

- What is Clinical Research?
- Types of Clinical Research
- Drug Research – a type
- Who are the players?
- Clinical trials – the parts
- Your role in research

2. What's in the Parkinson's Pipeline?
    - Understand the limitations of current PD treatments
    - Describe the difference between studies of symptomatic and neuroprotective treatments
    - Understand how observational studies help move PD research forward

3. Current Scientific Challenges to PD Research
    - Learn about challenges in identifying the causes of PD
    - Understand the difficulties in tracking the progression of PD
    - Learn how researchers are increasing their focus on non-motor symptoms

4. Improving the PD Research Process
    - Identify major barriers that can delay PD research studies
    - Understand the informed consent process and identify ways it can be improved

Learn what you can do to influence PD research and speed the development of new treatments

I am extremely appreciative of the breadth of coverage of the four part course. I feel I have learned so much about the complexities of PD research and of bringing new treatments into practice. I am especially appreciative of the research program that Pook has been signed up for and is about to participate in. However, recognizing my caregiver role for Pook, I fail to see how I can take time away, certainly not when travel is involved, to actively participate as a PDF Research Advocate.

CHAPTER 19 – PD/LBD DOCTOR COMMUNICATIONS AND A RESEARCH STUDY

Fax to PD/LBD doctor

Thank you for recommending her for the U of M FEOBV Protocol research study. We were both pleased to accept and hope that you might learn something of value regarding her treatment. The research team has agreed that she can take a tranquilizer in advance to avoid having an AFIB episode triggered by anxiety. The study itself mentions the use of Valium or Xanax thirty minutes before scanning in that regard. You had previously prescribed Buspirone for her anxiety attacks. I filled the prescription on February 12, but never gave her any.

My Questions:

(1) Should she take the Buspirone on the days of scanning, and also maybe the days before? The

drug's instructions indicate that it may take several days or weeks to reach the full effect. (2) Should I, or you, notify the investigators in advance that she should be given Valium or Xanax prior to any scanning? (3) Should her medication be adjusted in any way to try fore-stall Parkinson's taking over her left side also?

During the past several months her tremors have moved into her left foot in addition to her right foot and hand. These left foot tremors occur all the time when she is at the table eating; simultaneously having right foot tremors and bad/strong right hand tremors that force her to eat with her left hand (no tremors there). When relaxing watching television she has noticeable tremors in her right hand and, off and on, in either or both feet. While reading, she seldom experiences hand or foot tremors on either side. I am concerned that the let foot tremors are the beginning of her Parkinson's taking over both sides of her body. She still walks with good pace and stride while swinging both arms; but she tends to let her chin droop unless I remind her "chin up". We also go for 20 minute tandem bike rides almost every day or evening which she enjoys and does well.

PD/LBD Doctor Response

He recommends that she should have Valium instead of Buspirone and arranges for her to be given the Valium prior to the test. He believes the left leg tremors are related to her LBD and are not evidence of her PD moving over to her left side also and sees no value in adjusting her medication.

U of M Research Study

I bring the following note to the first day's appointment, called the Screening Day, for which they want basic background health information.

<u>Medications</u>

    Sinemet (Carb/Levo) – 25-100 mg – three times daily (8:00 AM; 2:00 PM; 8:00 PM
    Carb/Levo – extended release – 50-200 – Once daily at bedtime
    Metoprol – 100 mg - twice daily, at 8:00 AM and 8:00 PM; extra dose given when she goes into AFIB
    Donepezil – 10mg - once daily – 8:00 AM

Aspirin – 325 mg – Given every time she goes into AFIB

Parkinson's Manifestations

Shoulder stooping when she walks; tendency to let chin drop, unless reminded; but good pace and stride

Continual tongue movement in mouth

Resting tremors in right hand and leg; spreading to left leg in past several months; sometimes when lying on sofa; watching TV; not when reading

Essential tremors in right hand and leg often – especially severe when eating; spreading to left leg in past several months

LBD Manifestations

Personality and conversational ability have disappeared

Loss of long term memory

Difficulty recalling events of previous day

Confusion in finding her way around outside of home

Does not sleep well; cannot recall if she slept

Sometimes lies on sofa and stares into space for long periods

No Hallucinations or violent physical movements

Degree of Independence

Selects clothes and dresses herself

Personal hygiene – puts on and removes makeup; brushes teeth; showers; dyes hair; does nails
Makes bed daily
Washes and dries clothes
Vacuums carpet
Washes dishes sometimes
Limited assistance in meals preparation, helps with salads; husband does all cooking
Cannot do ironing because of tremors
Spends most of her time reading fiction daily

Physical Exercise

Does 30 to 40 minutes of "strength and stretch" exercises three times per week: uses a combination of 5 pound dumbbells; exercise ball; stretch cord; some yoga
20 to 30 minute walks through woods or on sidewalks, at least four times per week – weather dependent
20 to 30 minute tandem biking (really enjoys) four to five times per week – weather dependent

Mental Exercise

Spends 30 to 45 minutes three or four times per week:
- Recalling basic information (phone number/address; location, etc.)
- Memorizing poetry
- Spelling words forward and back

Handwriting practice
Note: exhibits good sense of humor
Also likes to do word search activity by herself occasionally

Vital Signs

Take blood pressure and pulse reading every morning about 7:00 or 8:00 AM; BP tends to be low – 110/60; pulse is medicated and averages between 50 and 60 beats per minute.
When in AFIB, pulse usually only goes up to 85-95 range; takes anywhere from 5 hours to 12 hours to return to normal; give her 325 mg aspirin when in AFIB
Breathing is always shallow and relatively fast

The second day of testing is the actual PET scanning which takes from 11:30 AM to 5:00 PM, with a lunch break between the two scanning sessions.

PD/LBD Doctor Communications – Fax

Thanks again for recommending Mary for the PET scanning research project at the U of M. The two days went well, including giving her Valium, which put her to sleep for both the scans. I hope they received good data. You, of course, have our permission, if it's necessary, to access any and all of Mary Ellen's data from the study. I hope it might shed some light on what's going on in her brain that might be helpful in giving you a better understanding of her condition.

Her right hand essential tremors have become severely bothersome the past several months when she goes to eat. She mostly ends up holding a spoon in her left hand and I must help her push food into it. I have been on the Essential Tremors web site and see that two different medications are considered to be helpful for most patients with bad tremors – Propranolol (Inderal) and Primidone (Mysoline). The Inderal, being a beta blocker appears to have similar effects as her current Metroprolol – decreasing pulse rate and blood pressure, and generally lasts for only about four hours. The Mysoline lasts for 24 hours. My older sister, who had seizures as a child, has been taking Mysoline for several decades for her condition and says she experiences very little side effects. Would it be appropriate for her to try a prescription for a small dosage of Mysoline, while still taking Metroprolol? Or, should her heart doctor, be contacted about possibly replacing her Metroprolol with Inderal?

PD/LBD Doctor Response

He provides a prescription for Mysoline. She tries it and it provides no help for her tremors.

CHAPTER 20 – MOVING FROM SUMMER ITO WINTER

The summer has been very busy so I have little time to pursue my year's goal of further Web research. I resume doing that research on colder days and find the following materials of potential importance regarding Pook's health situation.

Parkinson Pipeline Project

I find that the Parkinson's disease Foundation each year publishes a list of PD medications being tested in two categories – Symptomatic therapies and Neuroprotective therapies. Symptomatic drugs treat both motor and non-motor effects of PD. Symptomatic drugs already exist, but have side effects or are incapable of addressing certain symptoms. Neuroprotective treatments are those that will slow or prevent the progression of PD. No neuroprotective drugs exist and candidates are in the early stages of development, making their prospective use still many years away. The article covering the year 2010 includes a grid of 117 potential developments, covering four pages. Each medication is listed in terms of the class of treatments and in terms of where, in the four key phases of development, it currently stands, including the status of steps underway within each phase. Only ten developments are listed as being in the neuroprotective class. Of those, only four have advanced as far as beginning clinical trials. Three neuroprotective approaches are in pre-clinical discovery and validation trials. The hope is that, within about three years, a modestly effective neuroprotective therapy will be approved.

Studies of Dementia with Lewy Bodies

Unfortunately, I am unable to find any listing of research developments aimed toward LBD cures that is comparable to the PD pipeline Project.

Our Fall Activities

A highlight of the fall is a four day visit by my sister Addy and husband Jim; Pook's sister Colleen; and her brother Bud's widow, JoAnn. We have a great time and so do our kids and grandkids. We have time to talk a lot; renew our knowledge of each other and families; to laugh and joke. Pook benefits greatly, telling me every day that she is having fun. They are surprised to see her pedaling our tandem and to see how well she walks during a nice walk through the adjacent woods, viewing the fall colors.

Their departure leaves me with a lonely feeling and with some fear over what lies ahead for Pook with her dementia. I find myself walking around all choked up with tears in my eyes. She has lost so much in just two years. In April of 2010 she was still driving herself to play golf with girlfriends, five to eight miles away. She was diagnosed with Parkinson's and began taking Sinemet on July 6 of 2010. We were still playing golf. I could still go with her to our Metro Park in August. I left her alone twice, sitting reading a book on a park bench while I rode around an eight mile path for about half an hour. We bought a new sewing machine in September and she sewed valences and pillows, and we painted our kitchen/family room.

Here we are, just two years later. She seems so lost – knows she has Parkinson's and Lewy Body dementia and thinks about her health, but can't express what that means. She has had to give up exercising at our sports club, because they move to fast; because she became embarrassed at not being able to follow the exercises, being the only person with major health problems; and continually losing her way out of the locker room. She had so many friends, played bridge and tennis with different groups; made new friends with our new neighbors –

remembers very little of it all except their names and faces; can't remember much or anything about all of our travels. She very seldom says that anything is "fun". Her only pleasures are reading most of all day; some laughs when we do poetry and exercise. She watches the TV news; Dancing with the Stars program; American Idol; and interesting eight o'clock movies when we can find one. Best of all, she continues looking forward to our almost daily tandem bike rides.

I'm doing my best to try keep her happy, and to try keep her health from deteriorating. But despite such efforts, I worry about how much more she may have deteriorated a year from now. Winter will be tough with no tandem biking; outside walks replaced with mall walking; few visitors. We're so thankful for our daughter Jan and spouse Bob who have us over for dinner most every Sunday night, with grandsons Kyle and Tyler most of the time.

Our neighbors that we used to play golf with and exchanged some dinners with don't know how to function in her presence, with her dementia blocking conversation. Needless to say, they don't drop in or invite us over. A number of them volunteer to come over and sit with her while I run errands, or to give me a chance to get out for a while. I dislike having to intrude on their time and learn to take Pook in the car with me, sitting in the parked car for a short while, or depend on one of our kids or grandkids for such help.

Variety and stimulation are good for patients with Pook's conditions. She has lost the ability to play gin rummy with me anymore; can no longer return ping pong balls very well; will do word searches occasionally, but only if I help her. I'd like to try some traveling, as potentially being good for both of us. She's too nervous about flying so that's out. She doesn't like to be away from "home", so driving and staying in motels doesn't seem possible. I consider the rental of a motor home, where we would stay in the same interior surroundings each night; can do limited cooking; have your own bathroom and don't have to pack and unpack. We look at several together, but I decide against that option when I consider the possibility that something could happen to me and she would be unable to communicate.

PD/LBD Doctor November Visit and Communications

Current Medications

> Sinemet 25-100 – Takes 50 mg 3 times per day
> Sinemet 50-200 – Takes one 50 mg pill at bedtime
> Aricept 10 mg – Takes 20 mg each morning at 8:00 AM
> Metoprol 100 mg – Takes 50 mg at 8:00 AM and at 8:00 PM
> Primidone 50 mg – Takes 1-1/2 pills (75 mg) at bedtime for tremors
> Aspirin – Takes one 81 mg every day and an additional 325 mg each time she goes into AFIB

Medication changes and results since last appointment

> Began taking extended release Sinemet – excellent results; no longer wakes in the middle of the night with tremors; tends to sleep well until 7:00 or 8:00 AM
>
> Increased Aricept dosage to two pills each morning; seems to have improved her conversations ability with me – sat on the couch asking me questions yesterday while I was in the kitchen
>
> Started taking Primidone; gradually increased dosage from one-half pill to full pill to one and one-half pills; erratic results

General Condition

> I take her pulse and blood pressure each morning at about 8:00 AM. I detect an AFIB episode about once

every two to three weeks; pulse goes up to 90 or 95 beats/minute; give her extra 50 mg Metoprol plus one 325 mg aspirin; keep her lying down while in AFIB; episode lasts anywhere from four to 12 hours.

Still takes care of herself personally – puts on and takes off makeup; picks out clothes and dresses herself independently; takes showers; uses the bathroom; brushes her teeth every day. She washes clothes each week; does some vacuuming; does not cook; hasn't driven sine last year; can't iron because of tremors.

She reads constantly during the day; we go to library every week, but I pick-out her books as she can't scan the inside covers to understand what a book is all about.

She has begun to have occasional episodes of "freezing in place" when she goes to get up from sitting in a soft so I have to help her get up.

Still have weekly emphasis on exercising:

> *Rode tandem bike for 25 or 30 minutes 4 or 5 times per week all summer; she looked forward to each such ride.*
> *Also went for 30 minute walks on sidewalk or on wood-chip path through woods 3 or 4 times per week; good pace*

and stride; slumps slightly in shoulders; needs reminders to "keep your chin up", especially when walking through woods. Sometimes nervous so would grab my hand. Now mall walking 3 times per week for winter.

Quit doing water aerobics because she couldn't keep up with the pace of changes from one exercise to the next (none of the other participants had a health problem).

Have done "strength and stretch" exercises at home – including her work with 5 pound dumb-bells – about once per week during summer; now increased to 3 times per week for winter.

Limited poetry memorization work during summer; resumed more actively the past month or so. Still recalls three poems. Also includes work on spelling words forward and backwards; includes some hand writing of letters to friends.

Questions and concerns:

1. Her voice is getting weaker; I frequently have to go over to where she is sitting to be able to understand what she's saying. Should she undergo special voice training or use of a device she blows into to strengthen lungs?

2. *The Primidone provides erratic results – some days she has no tremors while eating meals; other days, her hands tremor, but leg and foot are okay. The tremors are worst when she tries to grasp something small, like a potato chip, or a piece of paper, but then okay when holding a glass in her hand. She has just been on the one and one-half pill dosage starting this week. Should she continue at that level or increase to two pills? Her left leg and foot tremors are still very bothersome, especially when eating; sometimes when reading; sometimes when watching TV.*

3. *In a book written by a medical doctor with Parkinson's and LBD, he talks about being able to think and speak better while taking Aricept and Namenda in combination. Would you recommend that for Mary?*

4. *She would like to visit her sister in Arizona for a week of two this winter. We were going to go last winter but she got too nervous and it triggered two AFIB episodes. Could she take some sort of tranquilizer several days before the airline flight to ease her mind about the flying?*

5. Have you learned anything of value from the research scanning program she volunteered for?

PD/LBD Doctor's Response

1. He doesn't feel that special voice training is necessary but he is aware of such training and leaves the decision up to me.

2. He feels that continuing with Sinemet at the 1-1/2 pill level is adequate; that increasing the dosage to two pills three times a day will not improve the tremors. Also, since the left leg tremors are most likely due to her LBD, not crossing over of the PD, increasing the Sinemet dosage will not help those tremors.

3. He does not recommend the use of Namenda; feels that benefits are not proven.

4. He provides a very limited prescription for a tranquilizer for the flight, if we choose to go, and recommends a trial of its usage first.

5. His understanding about the research scanning project is that the results will be published sometime in the future after all the data analysis is complete. The results are intended to be used to evaluate the efficacy of the chemical being tried and that analysis of individual patients is not possible and will not be attempted.

CHAPTER 21 – HER HEALTH IMPACTS

As we entered 2012, I was optimistic about Pook's health, that research programs underway might produce some worthwhile level of improvement in PD and/or LBD medication. In the meantime, Pook would continue to do well with the physical and mental exercises that we were doing most every day. Pook's health at the end of the year was, in some important respects, as good as it was at the beginning of the year:

> She was still quite physically fit, doing yoga, working through a variety of dumb-bell exercises, using stretch cords and inflated balls
>
> She has learned two pieces of poetry, and almost a third one
>
> She had begun to express herself, albeit quite crudely, with many mis-spelled words and poor sentence structuring, in some handwritten letters
>
> We were still able to go for frequent long walks; she maintained a good pace and stride

She was able to pedal and enjoy, the use of a tandem bike

She still dressed and showered by herself, and put on and took off makeup

She still smiled and laughed frequently

In other respects her health had deteriorated:

- I had taken over cooking meals almost totally

- Worsening of right hand tremors

- An increased frequency of irritating left foot tremors

- Her voice was getting weaker, more of a whisper, and her communication ability had deteriorated badly

- I was unable to leave her alone for more than half an hour at a time for fear she might wander off and get lost

- She refused to, or couldn't, play gin rummy with me any more

She gave up water aerobics for several reasons, one being her increasing confusion in finding her way around

Here's how she looked at Thanksgiving time in 2012.

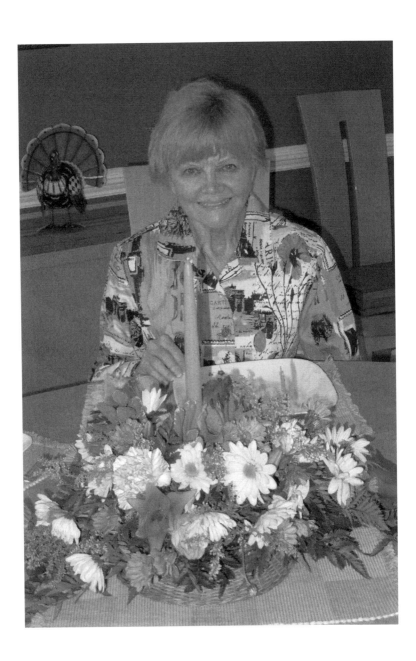

CHAPTER 22 – CAREGIVER LESSONS LEARNED

I began setting goals for important achievement areas – (1) research on possible symptom medication improvements or cures; and (2) improving Pook's communications ability, while also providing more mental exercise through hand writing letters to friends and relatives. Both goals led to actions on my part:

Goal One

I found an extensive list of ongoing medical research projects for PD, but little prospects for "breakthrough" achievements that might help Pook in the next several years. Especially frustrating was all the reporting of the prospects of an Alzheimer's solution from the cancer drug Bexaroten because of its immediate turnaround of symptoms on mice; a false alarm.

Goal Two

I was pleased, and proud, of her ability to focus and actually complete several hand written letters.

I added to my caregiver concerns:

> Becoming lonesome – As we experienced the pleasures of out-of-town visitors, then depression after their departure, with the prospects of the relative isolation of a long, cold winter ahead; along with the knowledge that, because of the further worsening of her verbal communications ability, friends and neighbors were reluctant to stop by, not knowing how to react to a visit where she was incapable of a two-way conversation and incapable of responding to questions.

> Experiencing an emotional roller coaster of positive exercise activities to depressing problems with tremors, seeing her speaking ability get worse, and finding zero prospects for PD or LBP improvements that might help Pook within a reasonable number of years.

YEAR 2013 – A SEVERE STROKE HAPPENS

CHAPTER 23 – BEGINNING DIRECTIONS

I send the following email on January 3 to a couple, good friends who we've traveled overseas with several times. It serves as a good status report on Pook's health, and as an introduction to our prospects for 2013.

> Mary Ellen, I hate to say, seems to be slowly deteriorating in little things – her voice has become a whisper; she "freezes" once in a while when she goes to get up from a couch, so I have to help her up; tremors occur frequently in her right hand and foot, and now in her left foot; both becoming very bothersome, especially when she's eating; and they keep her from writing. The good news parts – she's surviving my cooking! She still does a lot of activities that are carry over habits – putting on makeup, getting dressed, doing washing, etc. We go mall walking every other day and she still walks fairly fast and with good stride – no "Parkinson's shuffle". She gave up on water aerobics some time ago but we do "strength and stretch" exercises at

home for half an hour every other day, including some yoga and working out with dumbbells. She used to play bridge regularly with her girl-friends, but can't anymore, so we now settle for occasionally playing dominos. Taking down all the Christmas decoration, still with her help, was very depressing, as I found myself worrying about what next Christmas might be like.

We celebrated our 57th Anniversary on December 26. Then we had our second annual "Grandkids Party" on Dec. 29th – no parents allowed, and had a great time – I will have to send you a picture of the group – nine boys and girls plus one "serious" girl-friend. We play a game called "left, right, center" with dice; several variations of Bingo; a darts 'shooting gallery' I set up; and compete in putting practice, all for a bunch of prizes I assembled including headphones; cosmetics and fragrances; small plugin vacuum cleaners for their cars; bottles of Champagne; etc. Lots of conversation, heckling and even a little encouragement, all for a bunch of $20-25 prizes, with no one going home empty handed. Pook stays alert throughout, enjoying seeing all those grandkids in action, frequently telling me she's having fun. From time to time each of the grandkids gives her their personal attention, despite Pook's inability to respond verbally. We *serve them pizza and have a choice of several pies for dessert (store bought of course). They stay about three and one-half hours and we have a lot of laughs.*

Cross country skiing has become my twice a week respite here; using my Norske heritage, I guess. We have friends from Norway who have a "hytte", hut, in the mountains and live for winter cross-country skiing. They even ski about three or four miles to a little Lutheran (of course) church in the hills on Christmas Eve, and the church is only open then. I've been skiing around the end of our lake every other day (that's all my body can take) for about 30 or 40 minutes, with a lot of huffing and puffing, ever since we got our first good snowfall of seven or eight inches. It works out nicely since Mary Ellen can just look out the window and keep track of me.

We weren't comfortable with flying anywhere last year, but hope that we might visit her sister in Arizona in February of March, if we can overcome Pook's nervousness about resuming flying. Otherwise, our routines of last year will continue, recognizing that her communications ability will continue to decline, and hopeful that our physical exercise program will be sufficient to keep her tremors to a controllable level.

My Caregiver Goals, Actions and Feelings

Goals

I have the following goals in mind regarding my continuing care for Pook in 2013:

> Goal One - Continue with the same physical and mental exercise programs, carrying over from last year; the physical exercises helping to minimize the impacts of her tremors; the mental exercises slowing down further dementia deterioration from LBD.
>
> Goal Two - Escape Detroit for several weeks in February or March by flying to Mesa, Arizona to visit her sister.
>
> Goal Three - Resume searching the Web to learn about any further prospects for improving her PD and LBD medications.

Actions

My Web explorations quickly lead to the following new directions in PD/LBD research which offer long-term hope for breakthroughs.

Optogenetics

Ever since Pook was diagnosed with Parkinson's, I've been searching for hope from ongoing research that might delay, or even reverse, her PD symptoms. In January I stumble across an article from the National Parkinson's Foundation entitled: "Shining a Light on Parkinson's Disease: Optogenetics Has a Bright Future in Research". I'm immediately intrigued – will this technique be the approach that will get beyond just trying different compounds that could luckily become "the magic pill" cure?

The article defines optogenetics in this way –"The "opto" refers to placing light onto the brain to activate channels and/or enzymes that will ultimately change brain cell "firing". The technique is specific, and has the potential to add or delete firing patterns in the brain's native cells. Additionally, brain cell firing can be manipulated at precise millisecond intervals. The fiber optic light source can be mounted on the skull or placed deep within the brain. The "genetics" part of optogenetics utilizes simple virus carrier systems to deliver genes to the brain".

Optogenetics technology was "born" in 2005 at Stanford. It allows unbelievably precise measurements of what goes on inside the brain; what its circuits are like; how its internal communications functions; while also raising huge opportunities for dealing with flaws in the brain, such as Parkinson's. They've already learned much about how they might target certain neurons, or internal communication links to better control hand and foot tremors. Optogenetics works by inserting light sensitive "Opsins" into the brain by using inert viruses, and then triggering the opsins with laser beams to make things happen. (That's my ten cent summary of complex technology; try Wikipedia for a better explanation). So I'm hopeful that the learning curve can be very, very steep and lead the way to new Parkinson's treatments. I'm learning a little about universities working on the technology, such as MIT's Media lab, and look forward to keeping up to date on new developments as they occur. In the short time since Optogenetics was named, some seven or eight hundred labs are now working on the technology.

The article goes on to describe that it has already been demonstrated that optogenetics could either replace, or alternatively improve, an animal model of Parkinsonism. It also mentions researchers from Wake Forest using the optogenetics approach to control dopamine release. It concludes by stating "Activating brain circuits by using both light and genetics has thus evolved from a science fiction dream into true reality".

My Internet searching uncovers many other optogenetics articles including coverage in the Wikipedia Encyclopedia;

major coverage in a seven page article in Scientific American; another special feature article in Nature Methods, termed "Method of the year"; and a five page coverage in Stanford magazine called "New Light on the Brain". No time frame is mentioned for direct application to humans. Nevertheless, I'm excited for the possibilities that might lie ahead for helping Pook.

The Human Brain Project

I run across another article on the Internet called 'The Human Brain Project". The project is being initiated by the European Union as a ten year project with an expected cost of 1.2 billion Euros. The thought of over a billion dollars focused on overall brain research, compared to the few million dollars, or less, amounts devoted to bits and pieces of studies of PD medicine and cure possibilities, is mind boggling. The project is intending to be able to mine enormous volumes of clinical data, allowing researchers to understand the basic causes of brain diseases, a pre-condition for early diagnosis, prevention and cure, including such diseases as Alzheimer's, PD and LBD. Unfortunately, applicable results that could help Pook are at least ten years, and quite likely, more than ten years beyond their early targets for the project.

Feelings

I have lost the optimism I felt toward the end of the past year, when we could do many things together, enjoying her smiles and laughter - memorizing poetry, spelling words forward and backwards, riding our tandem frequently. I see her increasingly struggling with trying to express herself orally with brief phrases that I, in turn, must struggle to decipher. I mentally worry that Lewy Bodies are attacking her brain at a rate I hadn't expected, the basis for my overriding concern about a finite number of years remaining in her life span – maybe only two or three?

CHAPTER 24 – HER STROKE AND EXPERIENCING INPATIENT TREATMENT

Our routine continues in the same way as defined for November and December of 2012. I continue taking her pulse and blood pressure each morning; averages about 115.5/61 – pulse, 58. She has two episodes of AFIB, but her pulse only goes up to 81 and 85 beats per minute in those episodes.

A close friend and former neighbor dies and we attend his wake. She is visibly very upset and has an immediate AFIB episode, with her Pulse reaching 107. She has another AFIB episode just three day later, with her pulse going to 98.

We go for a mall walk on February 20 and she does word search for relaxation after we come home. She has another AFIB episode on the twenty first, with her pulse going up to 102. I give her a 325 mg aspirin and she recovers by 4:15 PM.

I get up at about eight o'clock on February 22, asking her if she is also ready to get up. She responds "not yet" so I leave her lying in bed. About fifteen minutes later I hear a thumping sound from upstairs, dash up the stairs and find her lying in the bathroom, foot tremors causing the floor pounding. She had put on her bathrobe and slippers since getting up and walked into the bathroom. She now lies slumped over against the bathtub; her right arm dangling uselessly, and it's obvious she has had a stroke. I call 911 and the emergency team is at our home within 5 minutes. She is immediately taken to our nearby hospital, Providence. She stays six days while they medicate her to prevent a further stroke and do tests to understand the extent of the stroke she's had. She also has to undergo a swallow test before she's cleared to leave the hospital. I sleep in her room every night. An attending physician stresses with me the importance of getting her into intense therapy as soon as possible.

CHAPTER 25 - MY POST-STROKE CAREGIVER ACTIONS

I look at options for her post-stroke therapy. I first try to get her into the University of Michigan rehab facility adjoining their hospital; they're booked up and will be for two more months. I visit another regional hospital's therapy facility, part of that hospital, and am immediately impressed – a big staff, and gorgeous "gymnasium-like" facility, with all kinds of specialized equipment for working with patients that have had strokes as well as other brain related problems – and they have a vacancy. Additionally, she has a private room with a couch that pulls out for sleeping, so I can sleep in her room every night, such is my continuing love and concern for her health. Pook is admitted to a program that gives her Physical and Occupational therapy, each for an hour a day, plus speech and recreational therapy at less intense levels. I'm told that the cost of the in-hospital program is covered by Medicare, for up to 100 days (100% for first 20 days, 80% for days up to 100). I am absolutely thankful for such a nearby facility and program within a reasonable thirty minute drive for access by our kids and grandkids. I have much to learn about the nature of their rehab program, and what results might possibly be achieved during her participation.

My Caregiver's perspective on Pook's stroke rehab services

I want to stay with Pook as much as possible, concerned about her ever feeling alone, worried about her stroke recovery prospects and unwilling to drive the commute of over 60 miles every day. I sleep in Pook's room every night. While sleeping there I am awakened each night by nurses and technicians who check on her, take pulse and blood pressure, plus clean her up if wet or dirty. I learn how to clean her up as she wets in her sleep almost every night. I get to recognize or become friendly with, many of the nurses and technicians, and am very impressed with their competence and compassion toward my wife, and toward other patients. Whenever I have a particular concerns or questions, a Physician's Assistant (PA) is around and accessible every morning. The head nurse also comes by each morning, is easy to discuss particular night-time concerns with, and is immediately responsive with actions.

Her daily schedule includes one hour each of Physical Therapy (PT) and Occupational Therapy (OT), broken up into one-half hour periods – usually one period of each in the morning and one period of each in the afternoon. Her speech therapy and recreational therapy are fewer days and lesser hours. I am immediately disappointed with both the speech therapy and the recreational therapy, but continue to take her to those, believing this to be the standard program required for everyone. Speech therapy consists of attempting to get her to recognize simple items, like hair brushes and pencils, and name their function. I already know that she is unable to do this because of her LBD, and explain this. She also cannot respond to the speech therapist questions, so frequently falls asleep for much of the sessions. We resort to distractions, such as candy suckers, to try keep her attention and to keep her awake. I feel that the therapist should be focusing on attempting to improve her ability to speak words and sentences more clearly. That, however, is outside of the therapist's standard program. The recreational therapy consists of learning to play a new game of dominos; again seeming to be a waste of time with her dementia condition. I finally drop both activities after a few weeks as futile, even though I'm unsure if that is permitted, or whether both are a requirement of participating in the overall therapy program. I do not receive any objections to my drop decisions.

I observe all of Pook's PT therapy sessions each day; respect how difficult the tasks are that the PT therapist pursues, and how genuinely nice she is. She is able to get Pook to smile and laugh from time to time despite the physical difficulties of the work. She begins by working with Pook trying to "get her centered"; using the balance bars, indicating that one impact of the stroke on standing ability is that she no longer knows where her balance point is. Just four days, she begins working with Pook on actual walking exercises, holding her up while she pushes Pook's weak right leg along with the therapist's right leg. Pook endeavors to hang onto the left side of the parallel bars, with her remaining good left arm, to help support herself. Pook also gets fitted with a right leg brace to counter Pook's tendency to drag her right toe as she takes a step. These efforts are unsuccessful in getting Pook to show progress in moving her right leg, because Pook still can't recognize the existence of that leg, let alone control it. Likewise, Pook is unable to hang onto the bar with her right hand, because of weakness and being unable to realize its existence any more.

I respect the PT therapist for the kind of effort she puts into her work with Pook, However, I am somewhat frustrated that, when she comes out for each session, she first pauses before saying "let's try this", like she has no particular plan in mind. Her PT therapy moves along, having her sit up and lean to one side and then the other, to strengthen her arms and shoulders; uses a "new step" exerciser a few times, forcing Pook to move both her arms and legs to strengthen them; and have her trying to walk with her weight supported by a sling from an overhead support, while she attempts to practice walking. The therapist also tries to modify a walker to allow Pook to lean on her right arm, rather than have to hold on by grasping the walker handle. The approach doesn't work. She also attempts to have Pook walk using a triangle support cane, without success. I find out that the PT only has two years' experience and I'm remiss in never asking whether she has she has ever worked with a stroke victim before especially one who also had PD or LBD, and I begin to have doubts about her stroke rehab knowledge and experience.

One morning I get Pook to kick her right (bad) leg up ten times in a row, until her foot hits my hand held at knee height, demonstrating the continuing ability of her brain to command her right leg to do something. Much later I will learn the importance of this activity so soon after her stroke). The therapist watches me get her to do this; never adds it to Pook's daily routine, so I still pursue it part time on my own.

I see another wheelchair patient doing what I term "wheelchair walks" along a corridor over several days, whereby he sits in the wheelchair and propels himself along by moving alternate feet forward. I start trying that technique with Pook as a way of again getting her brain to work at issuing commands to her bad leg. Working with her almost every afternoon for a week, she gets better and better. Unfortunately, I am trying this the last week or so before she is to be released.

The OT is the nicest person in the world, showing up first thing in the morning to help her get dressed, having extreme patience and speaking nicely to her all the while. Yet I leave Pook with this same person for several afternoon therapy sessions and she shows up with my wife ten minutes later saying "I can't work with her, she is <u>intentionally</u> shutting down on me (her eyes have closed)". I explain that, because of her Lewy Body Dementia, coupled with brain loss from the stroke, she is incapable of doing anything even close to such an intentional activity.

The OT concentrates on activities whereby Pook uses her able left arm, rather than trying to have her do any activities with the stroke weakened right arm. For example, she has Pook turning over and matching cards, using her left hand; also turning pegs over with her left hand. Right arm work consists solely of stretching exercises. The OT tells me that it is premature to work with the weakened right arm on any of several hand pedaling machines. So no right arm activities are ever done to try to stimulate linkages to her brain. The last week or so is just spent on doing various stretching exercises, to prevent spasticity, or maybe just because that successfully prevents her falling asleep.

I am very naïve, assuming that the resident doctors and therapists are professionals and know exactly what kind of daily therapy she needs, recognizing that she has had a severe stroke and, in addition, has PD and LBD. I have zero knowledge about what constitutes excellent therapy, so am unable to ask fundamental questions about the nature of the four different programs she is enrolled in. But as the days roll by, I become critical of many aspects of their work:

> They do not have, or are unable to communicate to me, what their plan is for moving Pook ahead, and what goals they are trying to achieve. Instead, it seems like they come to each session with seemingly, impromptu ideas, rather than any sort of specific plan; giving me the impression when they show up as just thinking about "well what should we do today"?

The Medicare constraints on her treatment are never explained to me, so I proceed to assume that Pook can stay at this facility until the one hundred Medicare permitted days are used up.

The attending physician that I see is a poor communicator. He never attempts to explain any aspect of her rehab program; each morning places his finger inside her hand and requests that she "squeeze", as if a miracle is expected, since no therapy is devoted to her fingers or grip.

I will forever wonder whether, if she had received great, or best possible, stroke rehab treatment, from experienced therapists, under the direction of a knowledgeable physiatrist, during that first month after her stroke - one who emphasized re-training her brain to command her stroke weakened right side - she could have made huge improvements toward beginning to walk and beginning to use her right arm and hand.

As we move into the third week of Pook's therapy program, I mention to the PA that I feel she isn't making as much progress as I expected and that I'll probably want to keep her in that program for five, maybe even six weeks. She doesn't tell me that such a stay is impossible. I'm later told that Pook's next step, after a four week stay, should be moving into a sub-acute rehab facility (having even less daily therapy). I respond by providing the PA with this summary of options as I see them:

Mary Ellen Haugen exit options

1. Exit sometime during the week of April 1 (a four week stay) – depending on sub-acute room availability and agreement with current facility's doctors and therapists
2. Exit sometime during week of April 8 (a five week stay) – depending on sub-acute room availability and agreement with current facility's doctors and therapists
3. Go home after four or six weeks, with staff therapists and social worker making recommendations for in-home facilities required; recommendations for in-house therapist and nursing support, or with outpatient support, possibly at another building within this facility, to begin a week or two after home therapy begins

My Caregiver actions required me to look at sub-acute facilities on the Internet and in person; to visit the out-patient building in this hospital complex

The PA and I discuss these options and I get continuing pressure to consider the option of moving Pook to a sub-acute facility as the next step, and she discourages me from considering the option of taking her directly home. I agree to visit a sub-acute facility, and visit two different such facilities, accompanied by my daughter and son. My goal is for Pook to get more, not less, therapy. The result of the visit to one such local facility gives me the feeling that it is nothing but a nursing home, predominantly with senile elderly patients having very little hope of recovery. The second facility has very little equipment of the sort that is needed to help with the recovery of a patient like Pook. I possess the drive and concern to have Pook continue to improve with time.

So I am especially shaken when, the day before the Friday marking our fourth week, I am told that we will be required to leave the next day! Apparently it had been decided by the overview group of therapists, along with the PA, and the resident doctor, that we would be required to leave that Friday, and arrangements were already in place for another patient to occupy her room - and no one had bothered to tell us. (When we had arrived four weeks previous, the occupancy rate was only about two thirds full. Now, for the first time in a while, all the rooms will be occupied).

I elect, against the recommendations of the PA, to bring my wife home, but on the following Monday. The facility social worker is on vacation for several weeks and the temporary one is of no help in working out what needs to be done when we leave there. The PA and social worker are also very busy and preoccupied with incoming patients who will fill all the rooms. Neither one seems to understand what the rights and needs are for a patient who is moving directly home. Neither seems concerned about whether or not my home will accommodate Pook - for example, how she will get in and out, having to navigate up and down our two condo steps; whether we have first level bathing facilities. The only assistance I get is that the PT therapist orders a wheelchair fitted to Pook prior to our departure. I am told that Medicare does not provide a hospital bed (they do). I cannot find out if any at home nursing assistance can be provided (it can't). I visit a local medical equipment supplier and they provide me with a hospital bed, paid for under Medicare.

At Home Caregiver Goals, Actions and Feelings

Goals

Goal One - When I get her home, and the bed has been delivered, it's obvious that a ramp will be required to get her wheelchair in and out, since our condo has several steps to enter. Our engineer son steps in and designs a ramp with the appropriate slope for bringing a wheelchair in and out. Another son, a son-in-law, two grandsons and a friend, spend one whole day getting lumber and building a ramp which is located inside our garage, so that when winter comes Pook won't be exposed to the weather while being loaded/unloaded to and from the car. Here's a picture of the ramp leading from our interior door through the garage to the outside driveway.

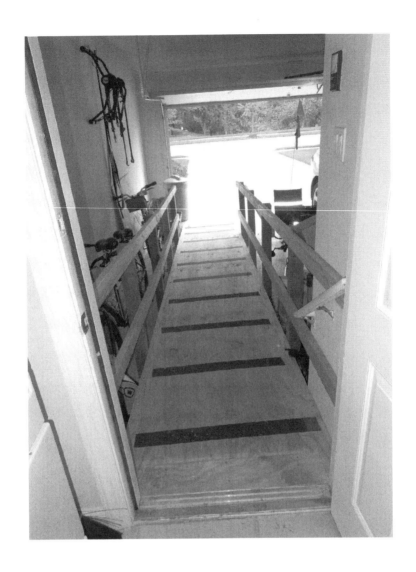

Goal Two – Locate some type of portable shower unit that I can put in place and then dismantle after each time I give her a shower. I search the Web and, fortunately, find a portable shower unit which, it turns out, can be custom fitted into a room adjoining our utility room where the washer and dryer are located. I immediately order it; receive it within one week; and find that it meets Pook's showering needs perfectly. It has a waterproof base area which is about six inches high, surrounded by light plastic curtains hung from round plastic curtain rods overlapping each other. I can wheel her inside through a curtained opening while seated on the wheelchair; wash her thoroughly; and shampoo her hair, using a spray connected to the laundry room tub. While the water is flowing in, a connected pump is pumping it out and into the laundry room sink. Here's a picture of the shower unit we found on the Internet under www.liteshoer.com.

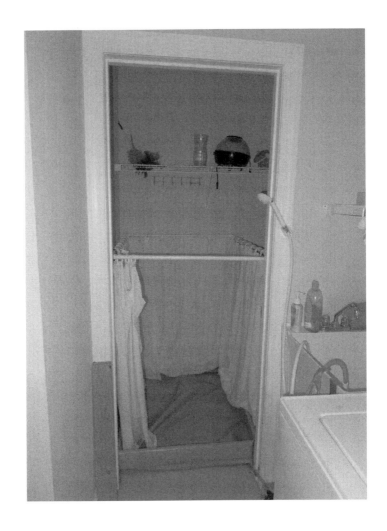

Goal Three - Find an outpatient facility where I might take Pook several days each week for continuing therapy. Searching the Web I find an outpatient facility only about four miles away; visit it and come away very impressed. Within two weeks I have her enrolled there and beginning a new program with different therapists. The facility, called RIM (Rehabilitation Institute of Michigan) – is associated with the Detroit Medical Center (DMC). I am especially impressed with their philosophy of encouraging the caregivers to participate in the patient's therapy, so time will be taken to getting me trained to be able to perform much of it at home. She will get both PT and OT services. We also meet with the speech therapist to ascertain whether she needs such services. After several practice sessions, we mutually agree that, because of her Lewy Body Dementia, speech therapy is inappropriate.

Actions

And so my long-term routine begins. Pook sleeps every night on the hospital bed in our family room/kitchen area; going to sleep between 9:00 and 10:00 PM. I choose to sleep on a couch in our adjoining living room, just ten steps away from her bed, and within easy hearing distance of any sleep disruptions she might have. Each evening I make up her bed with a waterproof bed pad, head pillow and foot/heel rest, and cover her with a sheet or blanket, as appropriate to the weather. I take cushions off the sofa where I sleep and make my bed with top and bottom sheets from upstairs. I also bring down the outfit I plan to dress her in for the next day. In the morning I get up about 7:00 AM, have tea and some light breakfast, and read a paper. Then at 8:00 or 8:30 I clean her up for the day. Every morning she is wet and maybe dirty. So I take off her night clothes and Depends underpants, clean her up with a scented spray and put clean underpants and undershirt on. I have learned how to tear off the soiled Depends, turn her on her side, and roll a clean pad underneath. I take the underpants and cleaning stuff some 16 steps down our ramp in the garage, always with a heavy sigh that that part of the day is over. I start the washer to take care of soiled underclothes and bed pad. I let her sleep until nine when I give her morning pills, before waking her and getting her dressed for breakfast at ten or ten thirty.

Feelings

The very last thing I do every night when I'm ready to go to bed, is to lean over her and say "Good night, sleep tight", to which she automatically responds "Don't let the bedbugs bite". Then I recap any nice features of the past day, before closing with "Love you Pook, have a good sleep"; our little ritual.

I very much dislike having to clean her up each morning and also additional times during some days, feeling bad that she has to go through this. But I won't even think about placing her in a nursing home where all of that will be taken care of by nurses. I am driven by recollections of all the good years we've had together and the knowledge that she would prefer being taken care of by me personally. As I clean her up I'm always talking to her, like everything is normal, telling her what kind of day we're expected to have and anything unusual we might be going to do. I'm also mentally bothered each time I go into her closet to pick out her clothes for the next day, seeing so many nice outfits she has always looked so good in, that I expect she'll never wear again. I also feel that I always want to dress her in a nice, coordinated outfit like I expect she would want to select herself; and never having her wear the same outfit two days in a row.

CHAPTER 26 – EXPERIENCING OUTPATIENT SERVICES

PT Services

We begin PT therapy on April 8, just eight days after departing the hospital based therapy facility. She receives one hour of PT on Mondays, Wednesdays and Fridays. Her therapist is impressive because of her experience level – some 20 years of PT work. The director informs me that this woman is her most capable PT therapist. She immediately begins work on defining the limits of Pook's post-stroke abilities. She works with her for three or four sessions on the parallel bars, trying to get her to hang on with her good hand while side stepping along the bars, with the instructor's assistance. She also places her in the "New Step" machine which has her simultaneously moving both her legs and arms to strengthen them. She also begins having Pook stand for 20 minutes per day in a device which brings a pad from behind to support her while standing; then does activities with her right hand and arm, such as picking up little bean bags with her right hand and placing them in a container, which is gradually moved further and further away. She has me begin working with Pook at home to also practice standing up. I stand her up next to our kitchen counter where bar stools are normally placed; Pook is supported by me with her strong left arm leaning on the counter; she then maneuvers different things around with her weak right arm and hand. The idea is to build up her standing strength in both legs, while also improving the use of her right hand and arm.

A little over two weeks after beginning the outpatient therapy at RIM, the PT therapist tells me that they are required to submit a written report to Medicare every two weeks, summarizing Pook's progress. She must show continuing progress for Medicare to continue funding her therapy. We jointly set two goals for the next two week period: (1) be able to stand up by herself from a seated position, although she can be supported after standing, so she doesn't fall; and (2) begin mentally recognizing her right side arm and leg. These are considered joint efforts between RIM and me, so they define an exercise program for me to do each day with her – practice having her stand from a seated position on a big chair or on her hospital bed; and have her stand for 10 to 15 minutes while leaning on our kitchen counter top. I also have her practice trying to kick her right leg up, and move her right arm sideways. The right leg exercise works only sometimes, but she is unable to command her right arm at all. Despite faithfully trying each day when we're not at RIM, I have trouble supporting her for longer than maybe five minutes while standing in the kitchen.

OT Services

These services are set at 45 minutes per day, also on Monday, Wednesday and Friday.

The OT, because of concerns about Pook's lack of recognition of her right arm and leg, has Pook place pegs in a peg board with her left hand, with Pook choosing where she wants to place them, then follows that with having her selectively extinguishing lights on a five foot square board. Both tests demonstrate Pook's inability to see/use her right side.

The OT spends a lot of time teaching me the correct way to work with Pook on ten different range of motion stretching exercises, to maintain flexibility in the shoulders, elbows, wrists and hands, for the purpose of staving off increasing spasticity or stiffness. She provides me a set of pictures demonstrating proper techniques to write notes on. Again, I take Pook through each of these exercises during days we're not at therapy.

The OT also spends considerable time with me demonstrating the use of an "Empi" machine. This machine, when leads are properly placed above nerves, provides an electrical signal which causes muscles to contract. I'm also supplied with a take home unit which I use daily with her right wrist and fingers, getting them to move in response to the electrical "triggers"; also her right leg. The OT therapist will continue to use her unit on Monday, Wednesday, and Friday, and I will use my at home unit the other days, so she has seven days a week coverage. I'm told that the use of the Empi unit is most successful if the patient also works to move her extremities in response to the Empi commands. I'm unsuccessful at getting Pook to do this.

I meet with her doctor from the hospital therapy unit, based on an agreement with the PT therapist, to have her right leg hamstring and hip muscles injected with Botox. The purpose of the Botox injections is to weaken those muscles, thus reducing their tightness (spasticity). We hope that this improvement will facilitate her straightening that leg, which has been hampering attempts to get her to walk.

Up to this time, I have naively assumed that Medicare will continue to pay for the outpatient services as part of the 100 days of expected services we have not come close to using up. I now learn that the outpatient services are part of Medicare Part B, with its own rules and limits for policy and payment:

1. The Medicare Part B financial support limit is $1920
2. The patient must, as I have learned, show progress in the bi-weekly reports submitted to Medicare

Our RIM services are, accordingly, terminated in the second week of May, due to lack of significant progress - so we are again on our own, an important difference being that I've received some significant training in how to work with Pook to try to make progress with her legs and arm.

CHAPTER 27 – DOCTOR APPOINTMENTS AND RESULTS

I meet with the same cardiologist that she had while in the hospital for her stroke, as a routine follow-on meeting. We discuss her medication, especially the issue of whether she should be placed on one of the new medications which have recently come out as possible replacements for Coumadin. He feels that the new blood thinning medications each has its own specific issues making them unsuitable for stroke prevention for Pook. He also feels that taking Coumadin is not a good option because of the risks of bumps and falls while under my home care. He recommends instead, that I give her a 325 mg coated aspirin daily.

Parkinson's Doctor Appointment and Results

We have her regularly scheduled six month appointment with her PD/LBD doctor. Here's a copy of my note to him:

Recent Medical History

> A left brain MCA stroke on February 22, 2013. Treated at Providence Park hospital. Moved to a hospital related rehab facility on February 28; stayed till April 1; then brought home.
>
> Began out-patient therapy at DMC Rehabilitation Institute of Michigan in Novi on April 15; terminated on May 16.

Current Situation

> Right arm and leg are weak. Right leg is somewhat responsive when Mary Ellen is told to lift and/or bend it. Right arm, wrist and hand are not yet responsive.
>
> Vision is mentally focused on her left side, seldom looking to her right. Does not recognize her weak right arm and leg.
>
> She received therapy at RIM on Mondays, Wednesdays and Fridays – 45 minutes of occupational therapy and one hour of physical therapy. She has spasticity in her right arm and leg. Majority of occupational therapy has, thus far, has tended to focus on arm, shoulder, wrist, and hand stretching exercises and on increasing visual recognition and use of right side. She was also

treated with an EMPI Neuromuscular Electrical Stimulation unit; I have been provided a home care unit been trained to use it on.

Physical therapy worked to get her to walk, a difficult and frustrating effort because of hamstring/knee spasticity, possibly combined with her Parkinson's problems. Also, the weakness in her right arm and hand did not allow her to hold onto a walker or parallel bars. The physical therapist was concerned that movement brings on "flexor withdrawal" due to her Parkinson's. Her hamstring and hip muscles have been injected with Botox and we found it did not make a significant difference in her legs spasticity and ability to function during exercise attempts.

Parkinson's related situation and questions

She still is able to recall poetry we learned together over a year ago, but recites it in a garbled voice. She still recognizes kids and grandkids; carries on restricted conversation; does not recall yesterday's events; cannot recall birthdate, age, years of marriage, locations, year or day. She has moments of lucid thoughts like: "Why do I have such a terrible life"? A comment made this week. She has been off Aricept since her stroke, until I resumed giving her one 10 mg pill daily one week ago.

Should I again increase her Aricept dosage to two pills?

Since her stroke, she goes to bed about an hour earlier and sleeps about two hours later in the morning. She frequently wakes but tends to keep her eyes closed; also "shut down" periodically during some therapy, closing her eyes. Speech therapy was impossible because of this tendency. *Might increasing her Sinemet dosage help in this regard?*

Do you have any general advice based on experience with other Parkinson's patients who have had strokes?

Current Medications

    8:00 AM or 9:00 AM –
- Metoprol – 1-50 mg tablet
- Sinemet – 1-1/2 tablets (37.5 mg)
- Aricept – 1-10 mg tablet
- 1-325 mg aspirin – (recommended by cardiologist rather than Coumadin)
- Stool softener – 1-58.6 mg tablet

12:00 noon-
- Sinemet – 1-1/2 tablets, except 2 tablets on therapy days

4:00 PM –

> Sinemet – 1-1/2 tablets
>
> 8:00 PM-
>
> Sinemet – 1-1/2 tablets
>
> Metoprol – 1-50 mg tablet
>
> Bedtime – Sinemet – 1-50 mg tablet of 50-200 dosage

PD Doctor's Response

Leave Aricept dosage as it is now

Her tendency to "shut down" is part of her LBD and changing her Sinemet dosage will have no impact

He is unaware of any PD patients that have learned to walk after suffering a severe stroke like Pook has.

He is pessimistic that it will ever be possible for her to walk again.

He recommends that I have her evaluated at a U of Mich. Clinic for what's called palliative care – to me, one step closer toward hospice care. Being a stubborn Norwegian, I refuse to accept the idea of her never being able to walk again.

CHAPTER 28 – HOME THERAPY AND AN IMPORTANT REFERENCE

My Caregiver Summer Goals and Actions

With both Pook's hospital based therapy and her outpatient therapy behind me, I now have to set goals for her personal therapy at home, based on what I've learned from the efforts by experienced "professional" therapists, and from what I've been able to glean from other sources in the meantime.

Initial Goals

She will stand straight in a walker for 5 minutes – holding on with both hands, without my physical support:

> Develop sufficient strength in right arm and shoulder; arm and shoulder must overcome tendency to withdraw while standing on both legs

Develop sufficient strength in right leg, while using ankle support, but no knee support

Right hand and wrist to use a grasping cuff with wrist support

Her general physical condition will be improved:

Pedal for 20 minutes with minimal motor assist on the RIM new step machine at least three times per week

Stand on both legs for a total of thirty minutes each day, using RIM equipment

Work on reducing arm and leg spasticity twice daily using the rented EMPI unit

Actions

I write up lists of therapy work to be accomplished each day and I'm far from sure whether she's capable of that much work and whether I'm capable of the discipline to follow my program plan day after day. The first week I am able to build up the time spent each day from one hour to three hours. It is extremely tough, far and away the toughest effort I've ever embarked on from a mental discipline standpoint. So I wonder – what if I fail; what if she makes some slight progress, but not enough?

So, I question myself every day – am I smart enough and capable enough to follow a program different and intense enough to achieve what professional rehab personnel haven't been able to accomplish, with what they've tried since her February stroke? So I look each day for little clues that might show I've begun to make some progress, and try to think of program adjustments to try the next day.

In early June I read a book entitled "Strong after Stroke" (by Peter G. Levine) wherein I obtain a critical overview of the nature and weaknesses of government supported post-stroke programs such as the first one that Pook participated in. I have, since reading that book repeatedly, become an advocate - every stroke victim and caregiver should be given a free copy when they begin a post-stroke rehab program. Here's a capsule summary of the author's most important points:

> He is cynical about the usual formal stroke rehab programs which he terms "meet 'em, greet 'em, treat 'em and street 'em". The doctors and therapists plans are to keep a stroke patient for only four weeks and then indicate that the patient has "plateaued"

toward getting better, so go home and practice compensation techniques to maximize use of the unaffected parts of your body.

He believes that there is no such thing as a stroke recovery plateau, certainly not in just four weeks.

It's a myth that recovery possibilities stop after 3 months or six months. Recovery improvements are possible even after five or ten years or longer.

Therapists are remiss in not spending any time on strength exercises for the stroke affected part of the body.

Therapists are remiss in not requiring many iterations of each exercise to give the brain time to re-learn anything. (They typically try a specific exercise ten times or less per day; the brain needs hundreds or thousands of iterations to re-learn previous functions.

Recovery must be patient driven – the patient (and the patient's caregiver) must learn how much work is really required to recover previous capabilities; how long it takes; and make a commitment to that effort. There is not enough time and money for a therapist to be at a patient's side for the necessary months or years of the recovery process.

I quickly modify my approach to Pook's home therapy, based on that book.

Revised Short Term Goals and Actions

<u>My Goal</u>

Get her to stand up from a sitting position, by herself, without my assistance – a major step toward beginning to walk.

<u>Actions</u>

The goal requires practicing moving from a seated

position to a standing one. Based on remarks in the "Strength after Stroke" book, my target is to achieve at least 1000 sit/stand motion iterations during the next two months to build her strength and get her brain to re-learn this motion. I start with her doing 20 sit/stands every other day, four days/week; a target of doing 40 per day by the next week, to get to 1000 tries by year-end. She's also doing ankle weight resistance exercises (kick-ups) with her weak right leg and hip – 180 in her first week; targeting over 1000 by year-end! I can already see encouraging progress with her brain responding - she can now command her brain to have the right leg lift up and kick my hand up to twenty times in a row – something the therapists never tried. A remaining big need is to build strength in her right leg by regularly pushing hard with it. So I start searching for the right kind of equipment to accomplish this.

She needs to extend her right arm and clench an object in her hand – the beginnings of eye/arm/hand coordination. Afternoons we work with hand dumbbells, three and a half pounds to start. New research inputs indicate that weight exercises will gradually eliminate the "spasticity" that keeps her arm held tight against her chest and her wrist locked hanging downward. We do 80 right hand weight curls in the first week and she is paying noticeably more attention to her right hand.

On the three alternate "resting" days each week

she'll be doing different "in bed" leg exercises in the morning for about one-half hour, plus I'll be massaging the weak leg and arm; add 15 or 20 minutes of electrical stimulation work on her hand and fingers in the afternoon on those days.

In total, my exercise program planned adds up to an average of two to two and one-half hours per day on busy days; maybe one to one and one-half hours on rest days. (She had been getting one and three quarter hours of therapy, 3 days per week in outpatient therapy). Is all this too much too much for a 76 year old woman who also has Parkinson's and Lewy Body Dementia? Or not enough for what her brain needs to recover? I feel that she is qualified to attempt such an effort based on her athletic history – playing tennis and golf; frequent walks and challenging hiking; skiing and biking.

If this "two month starter program" bears fruit, I hope, very optimistic ally, to have her walking by Christmas, maybe able to take ten steps; plus using her right arm and hand for eating and grooming her hair and face.

Additional Actions

I order a personal exercise device called a Weider, which has the user lying down on a movable support while pushing against his or her own weight to build up leg strength, working one leg at a time, or both legs working together. I especially hope to use it to have her push against her own weight with her weak right leg. The movable support is located on a frame which is adjustable in height, allowing the pushing resistance to be varied by raising the frame to a steeper angle.

I also order a recumbent trike, called a Terra Trike, which accommodates two persons pedaling at the same time. The lead driver, located between the two front wheels, steers, shifts and brakes. The person in back, located just in front of the single back wheel, joins the driver in pedaling through an extended chain. The trike is U.S. engineered and manufactured in China. The transmission can be shifted through a range of eight gears and all three wheels have disc brakes. The seats are recumbent and slung between pieces of tubing, like the seat in her wheelchair. I order a special attachment for her weak right leg which keeps it from caving inward and hitting the trike frame. My fervent hope is that it will allow us to continue to pedal around our neighborhoods, like we did last year when she could still ride our tandem bike with me. The trike is scheduled to arrive in mid-July.

Feelings

The "Strength After Stroke" book, which I read and re-read, gives me hope that, if I'm patient, and sufficiently disciplined, it may be possible to get her walking again and also be able to improve the functional ability of her right hand. I am also optimistic about the possibility of the trike allowing us to get outside in the sunshine frequently, exercising that weak right leg, while also giving her the enjoyment of looking around, to compensate for daily boredom.

CHAPTER 29 – ANOTHER CHANGE IN DIRECTION

Our Summer Relaxation Activities

With only her left hand usable, Pook is incapable of doing much; consequently she gets bored every day, making it tough to find enjoyable things for her to do. We go for two wheelchair walks every day depending on the weather; once a week to the library to pick out six or seven magazines to look at. She especially likes to browse through the kinds of ladies fashion magazines that she used to read – like Glamour and Allure. She will watch some television in mid-afternoon and/or after dinner. We begin using the trike and she has a positive attitude, liking to get outside, plus doing something similar to our past biking days. If we go out in the afternoon, she'll often indicate that she'd like to go out again in the evening.

August rolls around and our daughters throw a terrific party, to celebrate my 80th birthday and Pook's 77th. They invite current condo neighbors and old friends, including Pook's former tennis, golf and bridge partners; some 50 people in all. Two tents are setup to ward off the heat. They serve appetizers, wine and beer and most everyone stays for three or four hours. Pook's sister comes from Grand Forks, ND; my sister and her husband from the Minneapolis area; all staying with us for four days, providing great company for Pook, and you can tell how much more awake and attentive she is with all this company. I set up a large foam core display showing old pictures of both of us, together and separately. My sister surprises me with a quilt she has made, covering many aspects of my life. Pook's sister gives her a gorgeous locket, which I quickly fill with one picture of Pook and another of myself. Our one daughter had contrived to get a copy of our Christmas card list and had requested pictures and write-ups from old friends from other cities and states. We receive a huge number of cards and pictures full of reminisces about good times with all of those friends. After the party, we sit down and I read responses out loud to Pook and show her the pictures. She recalls people, and some of their names, but, unfortunately, her mind can't recollect the kind of trips or activities we have had with them.

At the urging of my daughter, I hire a "sitter", ("lady sitter" I call her) to come over two or three days some weeks, for two hours at a time, to give me some relief to exercise and to run errands. She is a college student working on her master's degree in social work; is very talkative and friendly. She and Pook get along very nicely right away, and I find that my two hour breaks uplift my spirits, if even just for brief walks through our adjacent woods or the chance to exercise alone on my bike at a nearby Metro park, or to go kayaking on our little lake. I find that I begin to look forward to scheduling "freedom" time. The importance of having time to keep the caregiver healthy is demonstrated when I end up having major dental work, having put it off for about five years, since before Pook was diagnosed with PD.

Palliative Care

My daughter urges me to reconsider meeting with the personnel at palliative care. She is concerned that, if anything were to happen to me, she wouldn't know who to contact at the University of Michigan to get some help. She would like to meet and know how to contact, a social worker who is knowledgeable about PD and LBD. So I setup an appointment, first sitting down and outlining what I would like to get out of such a meeting. I plan for my daughter, Jan, to accompany me to hear the discussion and give me her impressions. The brief note I plan to use as a discussion basis is as follows:

Mary Haugen Assistance Goals

Connect to a U of M Physiatrist for advice on coping with or eliminating spasticity; establish a link to therapists

Obtain therapist assistance:

    Long-term (6 months?) spasticity reduction exercises and definition of a functional program to meet a goal of having her walking again
    Another functional program, aimed at meeting a goal of being able to use both hands for a limited amount - eating and simple crafts
    Train her husband in performing all exercises properly and monitoring results

We meet with the head of the Palliative Care program, a supporting nurse and a supporting social worker. We have a good discussion regarding making sure that I have all documentation necessary in case Pook's health deteriorates further – such as Power of Attorney and Living Will, which we have prepared at least a year earlier. The social worker becomes the contact that my daughter is interested in, if something should happen to me. The social worker also assures me that she will obtain the physiatrist contact and link to therapists that I am requesting. Within two weeks I have an appointment scheduled with a U of M physiatrist.

Physiatrist Meeting

I bring Pook with me to the initial meeting with a physiatrist from the U of M Physical Medicine and Rehabilitation Department, providing him with a brief background on Pook's medical history, besides a copy of the note to the Palliative Clinic personnel:

He examines her briefly and I am immediately impressed with his appraisal of her condition. He works with a team of therapists and will set up appointments for Pook and me to meet with them during the month of December. He plans to meet with us again following our meetings with the therapist team members.

December Surprise

As I'm cleaning up Pook one morning, I notice that her right leg appears swollen. Looking at it intensely, it seems so much larger that I worry whether she could possibly have a blood clot in that leg. Fortunately, I'm able to get her in to see our family doctor that day and he is able to arrange for a specialist to perform some sophisticated testing on the leg to determine if she has a blood clot, and, if so, where it might be. The results are positive and she is admitted to our local hospital that evening. She receives treatment for the clot and is released five days later, along with a prescription for the use of Coumadin. Her hospital doctor recommends that her right leg should be exercised each day after she comes home, so we are able to resume therapy sessions with the U of M therapists immediately.

Follow up Meeting with Physiatrist

Results from December rehab meetings with therapists:

1. No apparent body of knowledge exists on whether it is possible to get a Parkinson's/Lewy Body Dementia patient to walk again following a stroke.

2. Post-stroke recovery for all stroke victims must follow six stages as defined by a Swedish doctor, Dr. Brunnstrom.

3. Exercise emphasis needs to shift from a focus on extending Ranges of Motion to one of emphasizing building Pook's voluntary movements anilities, implying improved brain linkages. Additional work needed to build strength, to enable her to stand, unsupported, for a five minute period.

4. Mary Ellen is currently in Brunnstrom stage 2 – with little or no voluntary movement of her right side limbs. Work needs to be done to move her from Stage 2 to Stage 3 over the next 2 to 3 months. Progress is to be measured primarily by the number and extent of voluntary movements.

5. Moving her from Stage 3 to Stage 4 will follow over the following two to three month period. Emphasis will then change to functional activities, such as: (1) taking first steps within parallel bars; and (2) her first feeding activities, lifting spoon and fork from plate to mouth using her right hand.

NOTE: Brunnstrom stages

Stage One: During the first stage, the whole bad side is completely limp. The arm, the leg, the torso, the face (including the mouth and tongue) are limp.

Stage Two: Spasticity starts to creep into the bad side of the body. Spasticity is generally considered a good thing at this point, because the affected side is no longer limp. Spasticity signals the beginning of messages getting from the nervous system to the limbs. Stage two is also when a basic form of synergies appear. There may be some small amount of voluntary movement available, but only within synergy.
NOTE: synergy means all parts of the limb move together.

Stage Three: During Stage 3, spasticity is at its strongest. Spasticity may become severe during this stage. This is the unfortunate part of Stage 3. The bright side is that you begin to control the synergies. This means that the limbs can be moved voluntarily as long as the movements are within synergies.

Stage Four: During Stage 4, spasticity begins to decline. In this stage, some movements outside of synergy appear. So, two positive things occur during Stage 4: Spasticity and synergistic movements begin to decline.

Stage Five: Synergies continue to decline. Folks in Stage 5 enjoy more voluntary control out of synergy. Spasticity continues to decline. Some movements appear normal.

Stage Six: This is the final stage. If this stage is achieved, movements look normal. Spasticity is absent except when fatigued or performing rapid movements. Individual joint movements become possible, and coordination approaches normal.

Why, when she was first placed in stroke rehab, wasn't the information on Brunnstrom stages discussed with me, and related to the kind of therapies she would be given? Because their stroke recovery efforts were not intended to achieve meaningful results? Even their handout

literature gives no clue about this important information.

My Revised Caregiver Goal: Recover to Brunnstrom Stage 3

I optimistically plan yet another home therapy program, based on these latest inputs from the U of M therapists. I add a wooden pole with a movable sleeve and a table mounted hand pedaling machine both to assist in arm exercises.

Right side specific goals:

1. Achieve extended Range of Motion
2. Begin voluntary synergy movements
3. Increase strength

Right side specific exercises:

1. Bilateral arm/shoulder stretching with clasped hands, plus <u>voluntary</u> wrist/finger work

2. <u>Voluntary</u> arm/shoulder, pole and sleeve exercises – moving the sleeve from right to left and across chest
3. Strength work with inflated ball – in/out and side to side motions
4. Leg exercises: Knee bends and lifts plus <u>voluntary</u> kick-ups and ball kick
5. Bilateral pole strength and stretch - hands together, up/down motion and hands apart – side to side motion

Mixed Exercises:

1. Voluntary wheelchair walk with legs while seated in the wheelchair(two times up and back); plus ball kick
2. Hand pedaling (5 to 10 minutes)
3. Voluntary Sit/stands from armchair – 20 times, plus six minutes standing unsupported

This is another huge undertaking planned to begin in January of 2014. It appears to be my last chance, working with these U of M therapists, to show some real progress for Pook.

CHAPTER 30 – HER HEALTH IMPACTS

Pook's health took a huge step backwards with the stroke, losing many of the remnants of her personality:

Immediately after the stroke, her daughters remarked on how much they could still understand her, maybe even a little bit better than just before. By years end, her communication ability had almost totally disappeared

At the end of 2012, she could still do mental exercises with me. Immediately following the stroke, she had totally lost those abilities

During her first phase of rehab, at the hospital, she still smiled and laughed quite frequently. Both had become rarities by year's end.

Immediately after the stroke, while in the hospital, and at initial rehab, she would follow programs on television; by years end was no longer capable or interested.

Her balance disappeared right away, and with it the possibility of again riding our tandem bike

Unable to walk, all thoughts of hitting golf balls were gone

Unable to walk, her life now became restricted to one floor of our condo

One "improvement" – she lost her right hand and leg tremors; though some left leg tremors continued

She became Incontinent

Her vision became primarily aware of her left side

She lost the use of two hands to feed herself

She now needed help to get dressed; could no longer put on makeup

As I look back at the year 2013, I find it hard to believe the roller coaster of activities and emotions that ensued, following personal expectations of a stable year 2012 for Pook's health. The totally unexpected stroke, led me into the ups and downs of five different sets of goals, actions and emotions as my knowledge of stroke rehab evolved – (1) hospital based rehab to (2) outpatient based rehab to (3) home based rehab one to (4) home based rehab two to (5) home based and U of M supported rehab.

Here's a picture of the two of us taken at the time of our birthday festivities.

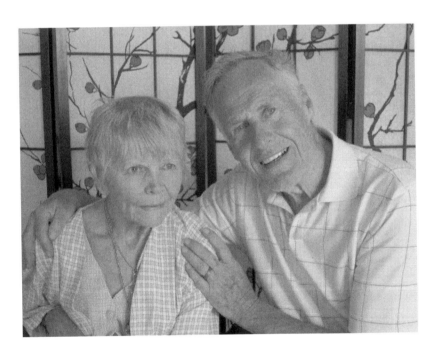

CHAPTER 31 – CAREGIVER LESSONS LEARNED

My caregiver learning progress expanded greatly following Pook's stroke, including the following:

1. Never give up on the search for new and better information. This dictum led me to find the book "Strength after Stroke" which so influenced my continuing work with Pook following her stroke.

2. The importance of planning what sort of program or programs you're going to be following for some reasonably long term period. I found that it was important for me to define goals; establish related action programs and recognize also my emotional involvement throughout 2013.

3. Be forceful in asking questions of medical personnel and especially, get answers in writing. I was remiss in not asking for (1) a copy of the first rehab program plan; (2) the experience level of therapists relative to work with stroke patients and PD/LBD patients; (3) why the OT therapist refused to work with Pook's stroke weakened right hand; and (4) why the OT didn't pursue wheelchair

walking as a useful and/or important type of therapy.

4. Always be willing to purchase new patient aids. In Pook's case, I found the Weider machine filled a need to help with leg strengthening (and I would later on find equivalent machines in use at other rehab facilities). My investment in the Terra Trike turned out to be the best investment ever for helping Pook with exercise and providing hours and hours of enjoyment for us together.

5. Hire a "sitter", who has a very cheery personality to spend at least several hours as companion for the patient, and for providing relief for you, the caregiver, several days per week. I learned just how valuable those few hours of freedom became over the course of a year or more.

6. Patience, patience, patience – I learned how much of a commitment it takes to attempt hundreds of repetitions of an exercise with very little to show for it, until you are surprised one day when everything all of a sudden seems to click. In my case, a thumb finally beginning to move in response to Pook's brain command was a cause for celebration.

7. Be willing to adapt any program you're pursuing, as new information and understanding become available.

Here's a picture of us pedaling our Terra Trike.

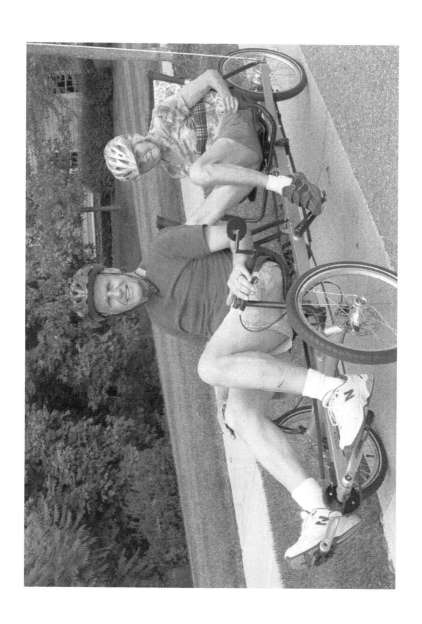

YEAR 2014 – A SHORTENED GOOD-BY TIME

CHAPTER 32 – A RENEWED OPTIMISTIC DIRECTION

I enter 2014 with a renewed sense of optimism. At the tail end of November we met with stroke specialists at the University of Michigan - a physiatrist (wonderful!); four meetings with an occupational therapist (sensational); and three meetings with physical therapists (good) at the University of Michigan Rehab facility. The combination of University of Michigan stroke related specialists - a competent and communicative physiatrist along with OT/PT therapists with a different perspective, has been a good end of 2013 learning experience. The result is a major change in emphasis for my exercise work with Pook – much less stretching to reduce the spasticity of her limb; instead, work on trying to get her brain to link-up with her limbs, through voluntary command of her muscles. They have taught me this:

The key to stroke recovery is awakening the link between the brain and the extremities – getting the brain to begin telling each extremity what to do, and then work to strengthen that linkage.

The simplest example of linking is the patient telling the thumb – "thumbs up!" – And building on that ability so the patient's brain/thumb combination can be repeated five or ten times in a row. Then endeavor to spread that ability to other fingers and, eventually, to the movement of the entire hand.

We (including the Doctor and therapists) have defined Pook as being in Brunnstrom Stage 2 – with a lot of spasticity and little or no voluntary control of her limbs. Based on their inputs, I've assembled an optimistic program plan covering the next two to three months.

My Caregiver Exercise Action Plan for Pook

Continue with a limited amount of Range of Motion stretching work

Continue with sit/stand practice, trying to get her able to stand-up by herself, including time spent practicing standing unsupported for periods as long as 10 minutes

Extensive repetitions (shooting for 1000 repetitions of each such activity over the 2 to 3 months) of exercises which gradually become voluntary including: (1) Move a sleeve about a foot along a rod with her weak right hand (and me helping) while I say "forward and back"; (2) Kick her right foot out when I say "kick my hand"; eventually kick an inflated ball instead; (3) lift her wrist and or a finger or thumb to do "thumbs up" at my request

Bilateral strength work lifting up and down a five foot length of wood dowel held in both hands

Aerobic motion work - hand pedaling a table top machine; foot pedaling our trike, indoors

My Caregiver Emotions

This new program represents a huge daily effort of two to two and one-half hours of practice. So we'll just have to see – do I have the discipline and stamina to take her through all this, five days a week? A huge, huge question: Does she have the stamina to tolerate so much exercise? I now understand that this is what it takes to recover from a massive stroke – mental focus plus a huge number of repetitions of commanded movements; even for someone who doesn't have Parkinson's or Lewy Body Dementia. Maybe I'm unrealistic or irrational to even try. But her physiatrist was extremely encouraging, telling me – "You are my hero!" His rationale for such a statement is my willingness to spend hours in home exercises with Pook. He indicated that stroke survivors and caregivers come to the U of M and expect the therapists to do everything. The caregivers then take them back home and do little or nothing between sessions. Furthermore, he added that for anyone with a progressive disease, such as PD, the caregiver usually gives up on trying exercise work in a very short time.

Physiatrist February Follow-up Meeting

My note to him summarizes Pook's current health:

I have tried splinting her legs some nights and have left them un-splinted other nights, and it doesn't seem to make any difference. If her legs are splinted for the night, as soon as I remove the splints, both her legs immediately "jackknife" back to the tightly bent position.

She has reached a point where she sleeps so much every day that I decided to withdraw the Tizantine (leg muscle relaxant) as possibly making that worse.

When I attempt to straighten her legs, I experience strong resistance, with her "good" leg, the left one, exhibiting the strongest resistance. When trying to very slowly straighten that leg I get a "ratcheting" feeling in her knee area.

She maintains a strong tendency to cross her legs all the time. When I have her seated in a big, overstuffed chair, I will place my knees between hers and attempt to slowly and gently force her knees apart. I can only get them about ten or so inches apart and then she shows signs of pain, so I have to be very careful with the limits.

I am no longer able to do "sit/stand" exercises with her because her left leg, the "good" one after the stroke, will not straighten when she stands.

I have been able to place her in our trike for indoor pedaling practice about once a week for 20 to 30 minutes; but she is very tired afterwards.

During January I worked with her five days a week on both upper and lower body exercises; succeeded in about 1000 repetitions of leg lift and kick exercises; 500 to 600 repetitions of six upper body exercises for shoulders, arms and hands. I'm extremely disappointed at my lack of success in getting her to routinely initiate any movements. Her best and only related performance was when she flexed her thumb only, for a period of five minutes; but never repeated that. I hope that her range of motion for right shoulder, arm and hand has improved some.

I slowed down considerably in my work with her in February - one week sidelined with a sore back; another week with dental problems, plus the leg spasticity becoming so bad.

Physiatrist Response

1. He is especially concerned about the limited motion problems with her left leg and will make an appointment to have her leg injected with Botox, and her groin area injected with Phenol, to provide

some numbing to assist in facilitating larger ranges of motion without pain.

2. He informs me that it is too late to hope for any spontaneous improvement in shoulder, arm and hand, despite the high number of repetitions that I've taken her through.

To improve, she must be intentionally involved in movement.

I'm emotionally distraught as it sounds like my focus on gaining as many repetitions as possible in a short period of time is for naught.

The reality is: she apparently has zero chance of ever regaining use of her right hand and arm; of ever being able to walk again!

CHAPTER 33 – A TYPICAL WINTER DAY

Morning

It's 7:10 AM on a cold Friday February morning in Novi, Michigan; temperature about 10 degrees Fahrenheit. (We are having what will prove to be a record setting bad winter in terms of cold and snow). I automatically wake about this time every morning, go to the bathroom, walk around the corner from my "bed" on our living room couch, and check on Pook, as I have already done two or three times through the night. She's asleep on a hospital bed in our kitchen/family room, just a dozen steps away. I take my sheets, pillow and blanket off the couch where I sleep ever night, head upstairs and get dressed for the day. A quick five or ten minute exercise routine and head back downstairs to begin the day's care of my wife. This has been my early morning routine for the past year, ever since she had her stroke.

I lean over the bed to wake her and her eyes are already open. "Good morning blue eyes. Did you sleep well? Let's get you cleaned up, okay?" I put on vinyl gloves and begin cleaning her up for the day. She is incontinent every night, so wears what are called "Depends" under-pants at night. I tear those off, wash her with a foaming body wash, and dry her with paper napkins; change the t-shirt she wears for a clean dry one; and slip on clean Depends. Sometimes she has also dirtied herself, so I say "So we've got a little pooper to clean up too". Taking care of that extra happens every three or four days. I roll the old waterproof pad from under her and roll a new dry one into place. All this time I keep up a stream of one-way conversation, or maybe even sing a few line of some song that comes into my head. She might answer a "yes" or "no" to a direct question, but otherwise doesn't speak to me. Finished, I always emit a heavy sigh; walk the length of the room, down our wheelchair ramp into the far end of the garage; drop the soiled underpants and cleanup materials in the garbage; and start the clothes washer going to clean her undershirt and pad.

I have a short respite to read my financial newspaper. Having worked for a number of different companies, and then as a consultant, I have a small private pension and have to keep an eye on limited stock investments. I take time for a brief personal breakfast, then it's time for her 9:00 AM pills – two Sinemet for her Parkinson's; a 325 mg aspirin for added stroke prevention; a 50 mg Metoprol to keep her heart rhythm between 50 and 70 beats per minute; plus a stool softener pill. She takes her pills in a spoon of apple sauce, with second and third spoons to help her swallow the pills. I follow with cold water through a straw, as she is always thirsty in the morning, caused by the relatively dry winter environment. I also feel her pulse to detect whether she might be in atrial fibrillation. I've gotten good at that, can sense whether her heart is beating too fast or not in rhythm. If I feel it's not normal, I will check more precisely with a wrist blood pressure and pulse monitor.

She naps for about 45 minutes after taking her pills, and then I get her dressed for the day, with an outfit I brought down from her upstairs closet last night. Selecting the next day's outfit from within her closet is always depressing or heart breaking – I look around at so many nice clothes that she has bought over the years, some which I have given her as gifts, and my eyes moisten as I see so many that in her crippled state, she'll never wear again. Since its winter, I assist her in putting on fleece slacks and top. She has always had such good taste in clothes that I dress her in a nice matching outfit, pointing out the colors as she gets dressed. I brush her hair, which causes her to automatically close her eyes for several minutes. I help her into the wheelchair; wheel her up to the breakfast table; clip on a bib and help her eat whatever breakfast I've prepared. Her favorite breakfast is French toast, made with sweet Hawaiian bread, topped with maple syrup, with orange juice or coffee to drink. She has always liked her morning coffee, purchasing "grind it yourself" type, mixing with some sort of flavors. I'm a tea drinker so don't know the first thing about making good coffee. Fortunately I learn from grandkids in college about a recent invention, the Keurig single cup coffee machine. I keep a wide variety of coffee selections in a convenient holder for her.

I let her eat the pieces of French bread with her fingers, messy though it is, since she always has trouble using utensils with her left hand. I make the French toast in triple batches, freezing several of those batches to have available for ease of use on other days. Breakfast is always an ordeal as she may eat two of three bites, fall asleep for several minutes, take a few more bites, and sleep some more. She looks at me and I try to engage her in conversation, talking about what we did yesterday, or what kind of weather today will bring. She might mumble a phrase or two that I usually can't understand, or answer a direct question, like: "Do you think I need to shave today?", but that's the extent of our morning communications.

Lastly I brush her teeth, put whitener toothpaste on the toothbrush; get her to open her mouth; and brush, using a battery powered tooth brush She lets me brush her left side teeth, but mostly can't get her to open her mouth so I can do a good job on the molars. To access her right, weak, side, I have to place one of my fingers inside that cheek and hold it open. Finally, I have her sip water through a straw to clean up her mouth.

I move her over to a big easy chair there and get her out of the wheelchair to sit there. I place a hand-made hardboard tray resting across the chair arms, with a ladies fashion magazine in front of her. She has always been interested in fashions and will turn pages and look at pictures. I sometimes ask her whether she likes a fashion shown on a particular page, but she doesn't seem to really care. Prior to her stroke she was a voracious reader, but, as typical with stroke victims, her eyes and brain will no longer allow her to track words from one line to the next, or even to read individual words. She looks at the magazine, and maybe dozes off a bit, before I begin her daily exercises at 11:00 or 11:30. I always have easy listening background music playing - bands instrumental music, or swing music which includes singers from the big band era.

And so our day begins.

LUNCH TIME

After exercising, we have lunch together. Lunch mostly consists of sandwiches supplemented by slices of apples and maybe a flavored Jell-O or Yoplait yogurt dessert, both of which she loves. Some months ago she exhibited some problems chewing wheat roll-ups, which had been our common lunch till then. I began making sandwiches with wheat "sliders", which are small-sized buns. The sandwiches typically contain small slices of cold meat – peppered turkey breast or chicken – plus slices of shredded cheese and pieces of orange pepper or cucumber. I heat the sandwiches long enough to just melt the cheese, then carefully keep watch to make sure she doesn't fill her mouth too full, and is swallowing every few bites. I also heat up some light gravy (au jus) to dip the sandwiches in to help her swallowing. She is always somewhat tired out from the morning exercises so goes down for an hour's nap, waking about 2:00 PM.

How to entertain her, and resist boredom, is an ever present question for which I don't have a universal solution. Today I pick out the smallest of her "magnet display "boards", one of five similarly framed sheets of painted metal, each holding parts off her 250 piece magnet collection. She sits in her wheelchair at a card table with cut down legs, which places the surface at a convenient low working level for her. I take the 30 magnets off the display board in front of her and place them all in a cardboard former hat box. I then urge her to pick them out one at a time and replace them on the board. She has always been meticulous and precise in every day household activities and this is no exception. She places each magnet in a precise orientation square to the board. We spend about 45 minutes doing this, including one or more five or ten minute breaks when she falls temporarily asleep. Each magnet represents a place we've been in our travels, or something we've done, such as a musical we've seen while in another city somewhere. So each time she pulls out a magnet, I review with her, what city or activity the picture within it represents. I'll never know whether any of this sinks in as she exhibits no verbal or facial gesture as a perceived response.

I then seat her again in the big chair for a second round of exercises; having just begun to see how well she tolerates doing two sets in one day. My desire is to speed the rate at which her brain experiences multiple repeats of brain commanded exercises, targeting completion of 1000 iterations over several months as a possible threshold for when her brain might awaken. I'm pleased with how well this second set of exercises goes; let her nap again afterward.

DINNER TIME

About 4:30 PM is time for me to begin dinner preparations. I took over all the cooking in 2012 when she lost her ability to follow recipe directions. All the years of her previous cooking and baking skills have made my job much easier. She had accumulated groups of recipes, by category – fish, beef, pork, vegetables, desserts, etc. She had also written a note in the margin on many recipes, whether she thought it was good, so-so, very good or excellent. I follow these recipes maybe 75% of the time; also have accumulated some other recipes from exploring the Internet looking for a particular type of meal.

I mostly make dinners made from cod, salmon, shrimp or chicken, along with steamed vegetables or easy microwaved rice. I also like to make hash brown or mashed potatoes and gravy. I purchased a wok a year or so ago, and find that stir frying is easy and quick. Some days I'm just too tired to spend much time on dinner preparations, so I have a number of quick meal solutions such as – omelets with cheese and orange peppers; various frozen entries; order pizza delivery, of course; or go out for a hamburger or fish and chips. I also make a recipe for pulled pork in a crock pot, which I turn into about three dozen slider sandwiches and freeze. I can then take out four of such sandwiches at a time and microwave them for a quick and easy lunch.

I move Pook over to the dining room table and leave her in the wheelchair. She is a good eater with a healthy appetite, but she struggles with handling utensils as they're now held in her former, rarely used for anything, left hand. I assist her in filling her spoon or in picking something up with her fork, but she places the food filled utensil in her mouth, I have a bib around her when eating because she also tends to drop a lot of food. A part of her eating problem is her lack of feeling in the right side of her lips; sometimes leaving her with a piece of food dangling from that lip. I must also watch that she doesn't fill her mouth too full as she sometimes ends up with a wad of food tucked in one corner of her right cheek, and I worry that she might choke on it. She drinks water through a straw along with her food and sometimes I give her a few swallows of wine or beer, which she still enjoys, as we together used to have wine with most of our dinners. Tonight we have a frozen Chicken Cordon Bleu entree, baked in the oven, accompanied by hash brown potatoes I make in a non-stick frying plan. I have a sweet tooth and entice her to join me in a cookie.

OUR EVENING TOGETHER

After dinner, I'm sometimes able to find an old movie for her to watch on TV while I do dishes and clean-up the kitchen. Tonight is a good night as we can switch back and forth between American Idol, a favorite of hers for years, and the Sochi Olympics Games. She is only awake and watching once in a while, preferring some diversions that keep her hands busy, such as searching our handy waste basket for folded cardboard boxes to play with.

At nine o'clock it's evening pill time – two Sinemet pills, one-half a Metoprolol and a Warfarin. She is alert taking them, but instead of watching TV, she plays with our place mats for a while and then with a string attached to the wheelchair. At nine or ten she says "yes" she's ready to go to bed, so I get her undressed and in bed. Our bed-time ritual is such that I place pillows strategically around her and cover her with her a flannel sheet. Then at about eleven o'clock I will "tuck her in" and tell her "Good Night, Sleep Tight, to which she mumbles: "Don't let the bed bugs bite". I tell her I love her and either review some fun things we've done, or visitors we've had today, or maybe tell her a little bit about what tomorrow will bring.

CHAPTER 34 – DOCTOR COMMUNICATIONS AND DIRECTIONS

March Fax to her PD/LBD doctor

Mary's current health situation has deteriorated over the winter:

> *She continually "scissors" her legs during the day, whether sitting up or lying down*
>
> *She draws up both legs tightly into the fetal position every night while sleeping. It becomes very difficult to straighten them in the morning; the left one (the "good one" following her stroke) will not straighten completely and the knee has a ratcheting feeling when I try to do so*
>
> *Her left arm and shoulder have gotten stiffer, hampering her ability to raise utensils to her mouth and feed herself*
>
> *Her previously robust appetite is much less so; she more and more falls asleep during meals; seems to*

forget to chew at times; I find residue food in her cheeks after meals

She sleeps a lot more, so I have withdrawn Aricept – which had no positive benefit – and also Tizantine, prescribed by Dr. Claflin as a muscle relaxant for her legs, which did not have the desired effect. Much of the sleepiness might be due to boredom, as she is watching less and less TV; shows less and less interest in looking at ladies fashion magazines; and has little else of routine interest.

When I take her out for fish and chips with family members, she is usually very alert, likes watching all the people there, and eats well with the fish and chips as finger food

I have continued to exercise with her for one-half to one hour most days, depending on her responsiveness – doing both upper and lower body exercises.

Her Physiatrist from the U of Michigan saw her on March 14, with regard to my concerns about her legs. He is planning to inject her legs with Botox, maybe as early as next week; and to have her groin area injected with Phenol, to relieve the scissoring, at the same time. The appointment has not yet been scheduled.

I have the following questions:

> *We have our regular 6 month appointment scheduled for May 15 – would you like to see her prior to her legs being injected or is our regular appointment okay?*
>
> *Is it possible to separate out what parts of her deterioration might be due to worsening PD or LBD versus stroke deterioration?*
>
> *Her PD medication has remained at the level of 2 pills three times per day. Is that amount still appropriate?*

PD/LBD Doctor Response

Her doctor doesn't feel it's necessary for him to see her before the leg injections; can't possibly separate out the degree of impact of each disease, or the stroke, on her health decline. He indicates that retaining her Sinemet at three times per day is just fine.

Pook appointment for leg injections

The doctor examines her and then proceeds to perform the injections, with no problems encountered; requests getting a report in about two weeks as to how the injections work out.

My follow up note to the doctor:

I have taken Mary through four PT rehab exercise training programs at the U of M Rehab facility during the past two weeks; doing exercises targeting extensions of her range of motion, following her injections of Botox and Phenol. The type of exercises taught by the UM therapists have been very valuable. I was pleased and impressed by their knowledge and ease of working with. Here's a summary of results:

1. When I get her lying down on a mat (I bought a 6 inch thick futon for this purpose) she doesn't lie flat – wants to remain bent forward somewhat at the waist, despite her legs placed flat. She also cants her upper body to the left, probably due to hip stiffness.

2. She still sleeps with her legs, led by the left one, bending sharply into the fetal position. First thing in the morning she complains about pain when I try to straighten the left one, which had the Botox injection.

3. Later in the day, usually in the afternoon, when I take her through the leg work again, both legs are capable of relaxing more, with some pain experienced if I stretch beyond comfort levels.

4. The biggest improvement has been in the ability to extend her legs apart. She formerly would not allow me to move them apart more than about 6 or 8 inches; can now have them slowly separated by about 16 to 18 inches.

5. The left leg will flex more easily, but still won't quite straighten all the way flat.

6. After rocking her legs from side to side, I bend them together to lie flat on the mat and press the opposite shoulder toward the mat also. Bending the legs flat to the right side is more difficult and she complains of pain when I push her left shoulder down.

She still tends to lean forward and bend down on her left side when in the wheelchair, or sitting in an overstuffed chair. You had previously mentioned that perhaps she should be fitted to a different wheelchair design that would maybe help in that regard. Should that be explored further?

Her doctor that performed the injections then recommends I contact the U of M wheelchair department about getting some type of wheelchair accessory strap to keep her in place while seated in the wheelchair.

PD/LBD DOCTOR May Meeting

My Note on Pook's health status:

1. General Health

    The extra bad winter took a toll on her health because of the very few times we were able to leave the house and the few visitors we had. She enjoys receiving visitors; still recognizes her four kids by *name most of the time; has trouble recalling names of all 14 grandkids.*

She has lost a considerable amount of weight. She was last weighed about a month ago and her weight was down to 95 pounds. Her arms have become very thin; she is much smaller around her waist and her bones seem to protrude more.

She eats just fine except that I help her half of the time because of difficulty using utensils. I also give her a glass of Ensure with almost all meals.

She tires easily, sleeps a lot and is mostly bored. She enjoys getting outside for wheelchair walks and I hope to resume pedaling our recumbent trike outside soon.

She has mostly lost her ability to smile and laugh in the past 6 months

She does not watch TV, says she can't follow plots or action; will sometimes watch parts of ladies golf; will watch some commercials.

She tries to tell me things, but I mostly can't make out the words she speaks.

2. Previous appointment with her physiatrist

    The doctor was concerned about her legs – (1) she sleeps in a fetal position with her left leg pulled up tight to her chest, and I have had difficulty straightening it in the mornings; (2) she tends to keep both legs crossed when seated, and I have difficulty separating them; and (3) both legs are stiff and difficult to bend. He set-up four hours of appointments with U of M PT therapists to get trained in leg exercises. He also scheduled an appointment with another doctor and had her legs injected to ease their stiffness; the left with Botox; the groin area with Phenol. We met a week after the injections and he was very pleased with her early progress.

3. Medications

    She is taking two Sinemet pills four times a day; no difference from just taking three times per day

    She is taking two Coumadin every Monday, Wednesday and Friday; a single Coumadin on all other days.

> She is taking a stool softener every day; bowel movements are regular; wets every night.

4. I am still doing fine health-wise. I have a girl who sits with Mary Ellen for two to three hour periods three times each week, so I get out for kayaking or biking exercise and to run errands.

Your Mom's Health – May, 2014

We met with her Parkinson's doctor yesterday for her regular every six months appointment. The results are:

> She has lost 20 pounds in the past six months and now weighs only 89 pounds. In May, 2010, when first diagnosed with PD, she weighed 132 pounds.

> This is typical of what happens to patients with progressive neurological diseases – they chew much more slowly and lose their appetite. There is nothing to be done to attempt to build her weight back up; provide food as usual and continue giving her Ensure protein drink with every meal.

He feels she suffers from abulia, typical with progressive dementia: a reduced interest in social interactions, spontaneous movements and in her usual pastimes. It also affects her eating in that patients may continue to chew or hold food in their mouths for some time, especially after having eaten part, and no longer have a strong appetite.

He considers her to be in the usual last stages of her diseases. Her body will gradually deteriorate as she loses more weight and will lose its ability to fight off infections, and so she might possibly end up with pneumonia.

He is pleased with how well she has done thus far with her combination of Parkinson's, Lewy Body and the stroke. He was surprised that she still knew her name, my name and could answer to being asked who I was with "he's my husband". He checked the movement of some of her limbs and especially noted the "ratcheting" effect of her knee as it's moved. He attributed that to the loss of weight also causing a loss of slippery fluid in the joints.

He decided that waiting another six months is too far away and scheduled our next appointment for four months from now, in September. If she maintains the same weight loss rate she'll weigh about 75 pounds at that time. Waiting a full six months would mean that her weight would be down to less than 70 pounds.

His only advice is to just keep her as comfortable as possible.

Physiatrist Meeting on June 19

I bring Pook along with me and provide him with this handout note:

Mary received the proposed leg/groin injections by on March 25 – Botox in her left leg and Phenol in her groin area. We had three exercise training meetings with rehab personnel in early April. We had an injections follow up meeting on April 15 and the doctor was pleasantly surprised with how effective the injections were in allowing better movement of both legs during leg/hip exercises.

She had her usual six month checkup with her PD/LBD doctor at the Movement Disorders Clinic on May 15. The results were extremely negative:

> *Mary was weighed and found to have lost 20 pounds in the six months since her previous checkup. Her weight has now gone down to just 89 pounds. NOTE: her usual healthy weight has always been between 125 and 130 pounds.*
>
> *Her PD/LBD doctor felt that her rapid weight loss was due to her entering the last stages of her progressive diseases, PD and LBD. He expects her to live only another four to six months. Our return visit with him scheduled for four months later, on September 18; a change from usual visits six months apart.*

Since her checkup with her PD/LBD doctor, I attempted to continue with leg/hip exercises as taught to me by your therapists. However, she increasingly exhibits pain when I try to straighten her left leg; attempt to move her hip in a sideways fashion; or to roll her onto her right side. So I have stopped doing the formal leg/hip exercises.

After some experiences with bureaucracy, I was able to buy a set of shoulder supporting straps that don't work for the wheelchair, but work just great when pedaling our recumbent trike.

I take her for two or three wheelchair walks most days that it's nice. We also pedal our three wheel recumbent trike once or twice a week for 15 or 20 minutes at a time. She experiences no pain while pedaling and looks around the neighborhood like she enjoys that recreation.

She still has a good appetite and I supplement her diet with Ensure shakes at each meal.

Her PD/LBD doctor's viewpoint (at least my interpretation of what he said) is that he expects her to continue losing weight until her immune system is unable to further fight off an infection. In response, I plan to forego further planned exercises and only do wheelchair walks and trike pedaling, and keep her comfortable.

The Physiatrist and I mutually agreed that there was no further need for us to meet.

I have another meeting with her PD/LBD doctor scheduled for September 18.

Chapter 35 – MY CHANGED CAREGIVER ATTITUDE

Emotions

I have now had meetings with two University of Michigan doctors I've come to know quite well, have the highest confidence in, and for whom I have great professional respect. Both have told me that Pook's health is such that it's impossible for her to ever recover, and her passing away is just questions of how long it will take and how might it happen. Ever since she was first diagnosed with PD, I've done everything personally possible to help her, holding on to an optimistic outlook, and suppressing thoughts of a day like this coming along. I am now mentally devastated! I want to go beyond "keep her comfortable". But what can I do to "keep her happy", when she is incapable of communicating what makes her happy in her present state?

The only answer lies in my daily choices of what we can still do together – wheelchair walks through our familiar neighborhood surroundings, with greetings from friendly neighbors; expanding trike pedaling tours which I know from last year, that she loves to do; more frequent visits from her kids and grandkids; and lots of little things from reading books to her to just rubbing her back, which she has always liked. But I'm also determined to make sure that she has adequate nutrition, and foods she enjoys, so she doesn't quickly wither away. I can already envision my expected depression when I will miss her daily companionship; and living in these surroundings with so many memories of what we've done together.

CHAPTER 36 – POOKS LAST MONTHS

July

Pook's health and appearance have changed much over the past several months. She pulls her legs tightly together while sleeping at night, then gets a painful look as I move them while cleaning her up in the morning. I have given up on the use of the futon for her to sleep on at night, even though I believe it's more comfortable than the hospital bed; her look especially painful if I go to lift her the extra distance from the futon. Her body has gotten so frail overall that it hurts me to see her like that. Her face now looks like that of a woman in her nineties. I struggle to stand her up as neither leg wants to straighten up in the morning; have to be careful to avoid straining my lower back excessively. When I go to feed her breakfast, she keeps falling asleep, doesn't then chew her food. I have to feed her, as she can't hold a utensil, or if given a muffin, squeezes it into pieces. So it takes me most of half an hour to complete her morning meal.

I fear that she is losing weight quickly, like her PD doctor seems to predict. I now weigh her every two weeks by first weighing myself, and then pick her up, a tough job, and step on the scale to weigh us together. I'm also giving her an Ensure drink with every meal, besides feeding her a milk shake every day about three o'clock.

I have been provided an at home device for checking her blood density, because of her Coumadin prescription. I received training at home on how to use the small sensing devise and how to phone in the results. I will be taking a blood sample, from a small pin prick in her finger tip, every two weeks, targeting keeping it in a desirable range of 2.0 to 3.0.

We have had such nice weather for the month of July that we spend a lot of time outside – average two wheel-chair walks every day; sometimes three in one day. We take our recumbent trike out ten different times and pedal all the way around our lake which is a distance of about three and one half miles; thirty five to forty minutes! Amazingly, that's about thirty five to forty miles we've covered! Sometimes we go out in mid-afternoon; sometimes after dinner, about 7:30 PM. Since I was able to purchase a "harness" which keeps her sitting up straight, she appears to enjoy each trip – looking around at the neighborhood streets, houses and flowers as she pedals. We also get a lot of people, especially those with accompanying kids on trikes, smiling and waving as we go by. I make sure to provide her water both before and after each trip, as she becomes very thirsty. Since she has lost so much weight, I also give her a milk shake – chocolate, pineapple, or peanut butter, after each of our pedals.

One morning I lie down to take a brief nap prior to getting her up for breakfast, and to get her dressed. I'm dreaming and suddenly Pook walks by. It take me a few seconds to grasp what's happening and I cry out – "You're walking!" "Yes I am" she answers, a big smile on her face; her personality back intact. "What happened"? I ask. Her answer, "I was lying there toying with the edge of my pillowcase, after our last exercises, and just decided to get up". "Quick, we've got to tell your sister the good news, and our kids". I go to dial the phone, still caught up in the dream, and instantly wake up. I've just been napping for ten or fifteen minutes and it's time to get her up. I do it with tears in my eyes and a desperate longing in my heart. The vivid nature of the vision in this dream will linger with me for over a week, bringing tears whenever it comes back to mind; recalling her as she used to be! While awake, all I can do is look at pictures of her, as she looked back when, but can't recall the personality details that went along with it.

I miss so much the opportunity that she and I had laughed about as we turned into our seventies, and had looked forward to someday, when we would sit in our rockers and laugh. I wish we could be able to sit and look at all the so many pictures we took as we traveled; be able to ask her: "How much do you remember about such and such, way back when we were dating? Or, about that skiing trip we took somewhere? Or about a river, or ocean, cruise that we took"? Most of all, I will forever yearn to see her smile again, and, hear her laugh, like she used to so often.

Here's she's being given an afternoon milk shake by Maddy, her wonderful, forever cheery, "sitter/companion":

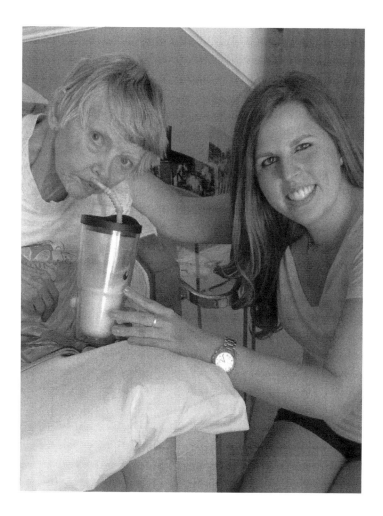

August

I have become so sensitive to the thought of losing her, that I look for chances to "keep her happy", as I interpret what that might mean to her. Each day I take her out for several wheel-chair walks; pedal our trike together every day or evening that is a reasonable temperature. She has nothing to do in the evenings after we go for a walk, or if we don't pedal our trike. So we sit on our outside deck to watch boats go by; or she just looks around. I will feed her yogurt or even place a dish of nuts in front of her which she picks at, and I share sips of light beer.

Nothing I find on television interest her at all. I will occasionally watch pieces of some shows, while she toys with place mats, an old wrist watch or such. I rub her back, which she always likes and talk to her about the day, looking into her eyes now and then. It's very personal, and I have thoughts of how much I'm going to miss having her around, even with her poor health and lack of ability to respond back to me.

August is the month of our birthdays, so talk to our siblings about some small get together around that time. Last year we had such a big party as I turned eighty and Pook turned 77, with relatives coming from the Midwest just for the occasion. I want to assemble the entire family in a last reunion, including all the grandkids and "their significant others", to have a picture taken of all of us together, something we've not done for years. But, with our son, Jimmy, having his blood cancer flare up, requiring new hospital treatment, and many of the grandkids headed for the fall term at colleges away, I find it impossible to achieve; so settle for getting individual families together for picture with Pook and I.

Saturday, the tenth is a good day, with the temperature in the high seventies and a nice breeze. I take Pook through morning arm and leg exercises just to keep her limber, but also for a bit of fun. I roll a large inflated ball up against her "good" left leg; push her foot tight against it; then push her lower leg out and say "kick it!" The ball rolls forward about two or three feet and I stop it. We do this some 15 times with each foot, and I let the ball roll out of my reach a number of times, a game she seems to like.

We are invited to our son, Leigh's house for a barbecue lunch. All four of their kids are there, a last get together before they all leave for college next week. Pook has a cheeseburger and sips on a glass of beer, periodically reaching out to take the beer glass for another sip. She is sometimes awake; sometimes napping. When awake she will stare at one or more of her grandkids whom she hasn't seen much all summer. We have key lime pie and she enjoys getting her fingers in it, then licking her fingers. We stay two hours, even though I forgot to bring her Sinemet pills, and have nice conversations with our grandkids.

That evening we take out our trike to pedal around the neighborhood. It's a beautiful evening and we pedal for almost an hour. Part way along I ask her - "Are you doing okay?" She surprisingly responds, loud enough for me to hear up front – Yes, I'm doing just fine!" Upon our return we sit out on the deck and have chocolate ice cream sundaes.

I'm so pleased how I'm still able to do some things with Pook that she still enjoys; not like she has Alzheimer's. She still knows me. She still responds to questions, though mainly with yes and no answers. We can still share pedaling our trike with her enjoying looking around; share kicking the ball; share having ice cream; share a few words now and then. I'd just as soon that she "slipped away" doing things like that, without pain and suffering; leaving memories of these "fun" thing done together on a nice day in late summer.

Our daughter takes our picture together on her birthday. She is holding a pink stuffed teddy bear that he granddaughter, Hannah, had thoughtfully given her.

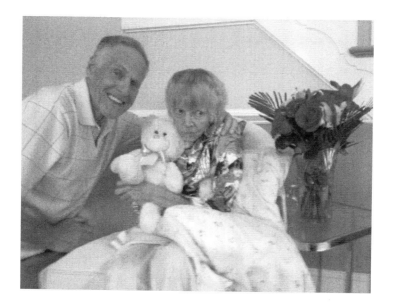

September

The early days of the month provide nice weather – many warm and sunny days, yet cool nights for sleeping. We get out for two wheelchair walks most days and for trike pedals four times. We also have dinner out on our deck several times; sit and watch silent electric powered pontoon boats go by until darkness sets in. But the middles of the month days turn cold and rainy, keeping us in the house; worrying about the onset of winter and its confines.

She comes down with a urinary infection which doesn't respond to an initial regimen of antibiotics; sets me worrying about her weakening immune systems. We have a regular appointment with her PD/LBD doctor on September 18. Here is a copy of my note to him, and his response.

PD/LBD Doctor, reference Mary Haugen:

We last met on May 15 at which time you were very concerned about Mary's weight loss over the winter (losing some 20 pounds, and then down to 89 pounds), and that her health was entering a phase termed Abulia. Here's her heath status since then:

1. We have had a wonderful summer!

    a. Her weight has stayed essentially constant at 87-88 pounds (while wearing shorts all summer). (I weigh her every two weeks).

    b. We go out pedaling our Terra Trike about two to three times per week; for four miles on the average; a total of about 30 times to date, or near 120 miles; taking 40 minutes each time. She loves doing that and looks forward to it. Her shoulders are supported by a "harness" which keeps her seated upright, allowing her to look around to both sides as she pedals along with me.

c. Her appetite has remained excellent. She normally takes big bites of food offered to her; but eats less in total at each seating. I feed her some foods; other times I fill a fork or spoon and she will take it and feed herself. She chews vigorously without any pressure from me and swallows just fine. She gets an Ensure drink at most meals and milk shakes or root beer floats in the middle of most afternoons.

d. She still retains an interested "spark of life", enjoying wheelchair walks twice per day; exercises involving kicking an inflatable ball; our trike rides; turning the pages of ladies style magazines; any get togethers with family and when having special treats, such as milk shakes, root beer floats and apple turnovers.

e. She remains responsive to questions – answering "yes" or "no" frequently; also repeating an answer to alternatives such as "Do you want to stay up or go to bed"? She will say "I want to go to bed".

2. She still sleeps in a tightly folded position

   a. Her legs exhibit a ratcheting feeling as I work to unfold her in the morning; shows a brief pained look on her face

   b. She is incontinent every night; defecates quite regularly

   c. She will straighten her right leg sufficiently to stand somewhat, but her left leg will not straighten

   d. She continues to cross her legs, despite having a phenol injection several months ago

   e. She sleeps a lot and will often fall asleep, or at least close her eyes, during a meal

   f. She tends to sag forward at the hips and neck while seated in a big chair or the wheelchair. I often put on a soft padded neck brace, which helps support her neck; it also seems to keep her more alert and she doesn't seem to mind it being on.

3. Medication

    a. She has been taking two 25-100 mg Sinemet, four times a day for about the last six months.
    b. She takes Coumadin, two 2 mg pills on M, W and F; one pill on other days
    c. She takes one 50 mg Metoprolol each morning and at bedtime

Concerns

She had a choking episode about a month ago. I called 911 since her lips were turning blue. No cause was found; but she was also found to have a urinary infection. She took an antibiotic (I failed to record the name of it), four pills per day for one week, to try it clear it up. A urine sample afterwards showed that she still had the infection. Her family doctor has now placed her on a stronger antibiotic, Cephalexin 500 mg, for ten days, plus a 325 mg aspirin. She also has a small bed sore that I am medicating. So I am very concerned that either or both of these could be indications of her weakening immune system.

I also notice that her always very thick hair is slowly thinning out, with strands coming out on a comb every morning.

Doctor Response

Her PD/LBD doctor is very pleased with how alert she is; that her weight has been maintained at 87-88 pounds ever since last winter; and she still has a good appetite. Most importantly, he talks about the value of our trike rides, wheelchair walks and other exercises that together provide such a healthy and enjoyable stimulus. He provides the opinion that without that stimulus, she wouldn't have survived until today's appointment. I briefly express my concern about the restricted opportunities for stimulus during the winter months which, I feel, led to her huge weight loss through last year's long, tough winter. He stresses how important continuing sources of stimulus are to her continued alertness and interest in life. the pills he can prescribe are a much less important factor in her survival.

I am relieved and optimistic following my meeting with her PD/LBD doctor, learning of his feelings about the value of exercise and stimulation in her life. I leave the meeting feeling (1) that a good chance exists that we – I and the family –can reasonably expect Pook to still be with us to once again enjoy Christmas; and (2) that I need to look into the possibilities of somehow getting Pook, along with our beloved Terra Trike, somewhere down south – perhaps Florida or Arizona – for some portion or portions of the winter beyond Christmas, to try to extend the variety of outdoor stimulations we've enjoyed so much throughout this summer.

Book Closure – for now

My Prologue expressed hope that medical research might have come up with a cure for her Parkinson's disease, and/or her Lewy Body Dementia, by this time. That has not happened. Neither does any timely hope exist for medications that might reverse either of her progressive diseases, or even delay their progression.

Pook and I continue enjoying a lot of little things together:

> Wheelchair walks and pedaling our trike together in the sunshine; kicking an inflated ball or pushing against it with her hands

Conversations, overwhelming one-way, about the weather, what we did yesterday, what we we'll do today, etc. She sometimes mumbles a response, but just her presence seems important enough

I provide her women's style magazines which we'll periodically page through together; my opinions expressed, based on what I recall about the nature of her tastes in clothes, in the way of having a conversation

I'll watch part of a TV program and rub her back as she plays with placemats, looking up at me, maybe tugging at my shirt occasionally

I'll go to the grocery store and she'll say she wants to join me inside, some pleasure in watching the other shoppers

Family members, and grandkids, visit and she enjoys their companionship, or we meet for fish and chips at a local bar where she likes looking around at people

We share an afternoon treat – a milk shake, root beer float, a coffee cake I baked or apple or cherry turnovers from the grocery store

I have learned through my almost five years of experience with Pook, the huge importance of the role that a caregiver can play! I feel the pressure of continuing to persist in daily caregiver tasks and yet to conceive of innovative ideas for the expected long dark days of winter. I dread the lonesome feeling I know will exist after she's gone.

I will continue to add additional information about Pook and my caregiving through the months to come, through a blog, or through periodic book updates to this book.

The day will come when she leaves us - then I will complete this book.

Made in the USA
San Bernardino, CA
18 November 2014